Heaven Can Wait
Surviving Cancer

Charlie Jones
Kim Doren

SEVEN LOCKS PRESS

Santa Ana, California

Library of Congress Cataloging-in-Publication Data is available from the publisher.
ISBN 1-931643-26-1

Book design by Heather Buchman
Cover photo by Kim Doren
Author's photo by Michael Loftus

Dedication

*H*eaven Can Wait: Surviving Cancer is dedicated to all the men and women who have pledged their lives to finding a cure for cancer. Cancer can go into remission but, as of now, cannot be cured. So from all cancer survivors and their loved ones, here is our wish—hurry.

Table of Contents

Foreword by Richard Hall, M.D., F.A.C.S. ix

Introduction xi

CHAPTER 1   The State of Cancer 1

CHAPTER 2   Coping with Cancer 20

CHAPTER 3   Kids Are Tough 63

CHAPTER 4   Women's Choice 97

CHAPTER 5   Largest Men's Club in America 131

CHAPTER 6   Attitude-Attitude-Attitude 168

The Last Word 190

Cancer Camp Directory 191

Index 192

Foreword

Heaven Can Wait: Surviving Cancer is a story that needs to be told. There's variability in response to cancer treatment from patient to patient, just as there is variability in treatments from surgeon to radiotherapist to medical oncologist.

The patients who do the best are the ones who commit themselves to the idea that they're going to have a period of discomfort, whether it's because of surgery, radiation, or chemo, but it will ultimately get better. All of the fatigue factors are real, but they vary from person to person. During the first three to four months after treatment is when there is the greatest price to pay in terms of energy loss.

It's all in the eyes of the beholder; everyone looks at things differently. This is truly an interesting subject because cancer, in one form or another, has touched all of us; and cancer patients and their families and friends need to know how other patients have reacted to what they've been experiencing.

— Richard Hall, M.D., F.A.C.S.,
  Urologic surgeon specializing in
  surgical oncology, Diplomate of the
  American Board of Urology

Introduction

Charlie

My journey started in December of 2001 when my urologist noted that my PSA was creeping higher, up to 8.70; after an exam and biopsy and a Gleason score of 6, he gave me the really bad news. I had prostate cancer. My first reaction was, "Why me?"

As a male over fifty, I know I'm a prime candidate for prostate cancer, perhaps the biggest men's club in America. Plus, I know that if you're a man who's going to have cancer, the two "best" kinds to have are skin and prostate. But it's still cancer, it's still the "Big C," and it's still a part of the alphabet with which I really don't want to be associated. Prostate cancer will kill 31,500 American men this year. So, I had to ask, "Will I die?"

My first option was surgery because there's a better chance of getting all the cancer with this procedure. However, at age seventy-one, my cardiologist didn't think my heart was strong enough to withstand a four-hour operation. And, after running all the tests, he diagnosed heart failure and implanted a defibrillator in my chest, eliminating any possibility of major surgery.

The next option was eight weeks of radiation, the gift that keeps on giving. I chose this route, and it wasn't a bad choice for the first five weeks, but then the radiation began to take its toll. It completely drained me of all my energy. I felt like an empty bucket. Some days it took all my mental strength just to get out of bed, walk down the hall, sit in the kitchen, and read a newspaper. (There was one pleasing note to the radiation; I lost twenty-five pounds that I had been struggling to shed. The doctors still can't figure out why. Radiation is not supposed to cause weight loss.)

I best describe my experience as riding a roller coaster. Some days I was way up in the sky, fully on the road to recovery. Other days I was way down at the bottom, to the point where I lost my enthusiasm for everything. A recurring problem was when I had two good days in a row. Hooray, I'm well! I proceeded to overdo it and then I crashed.

I began to wonder if it was just me, if I was the exception, if I was the wimp who couldn't handle it. I also began to wonder, "What's next?"

Kim

Although I have never had cancer, it has significantly touched my life. Two of my grandparents died from this terrible disease, and I've seen how my dad (prostate cancer), my aunt (breast cancer), my uncle (colon cancer), and some good friends, have all handled their battles with cancer. When Charlie was diagnosed, I thought one way to help him cope with his cancer would be to have him hear encouragement from others who had faced similar challenges. I suggested he interview people, just as we have done for our previous books, figuring it could serve, surreptitiously, as therapy. In doing so, we witnessed the tremendous courage, grace, and humor of these survivors, and it dawned on us—their stories should be shared with everyone.

Charlie

Following Kim's suggestion, I started talking with friends of mine who had had all kinds of cancer treatments: radiation, surgery, chemo, radiotherapy, arsenic trioxide, and hormonal therapy. I asked them how they coped with their cancer. I discovered there are multitudes of answers to this question, and they apply across the board. What a female ovarian cancer survivor learned will help a male who is battling testicular cancer, and vice versa.

Kim

We talked with cancer survivors from all over the country, in addition to leading cancer physicians and researchers nationwide, who offered their knowledgeable insights. From these conversations, we also discovered what may be the most important element of cancer remission and recovery. It's simply one word: attitude. When we understood that, we knew this was a book that we had to write.

There is still a lot of work yet to be done in cancer research, but great progress is being made. This book won't cure cancer, but through the power of the positive personal examples shared by these recovering cancer patients and leading physicians, we hope *Heaven Can Wait: Surviving Cancer* will help make life more manageable and fulfilling for cancer survivors, and their families and friends.

Chapter One
The State of Cancer

Currently, there are more than ten million recovering cancer patients in the United States, and cancer cases continue to grow at an alarming rate—over 12 percent a year; more than 3,500,000 new cancer patients over the last three years. Although there are ten million people "recovering," the fact is, there is still no cure for cancer. Even after treatment, cancer patients must learn to live with the disease.

Perhaps the greatest research discovery involves DNA and cancer cells, and the determination that all cancers are not the same. For decades, the main treatment for cancer was radiation and chemotherapy, which killed healthy and cancerous cells alike. But thanks to the unraveling of the human genome, scientists are on the brink of narrowly targeted, genetically geared therapies tailored to a specific patient's cancer.

The future portends a complete new style of cancer treatments, such as customized cancer cocktails whose recipes are determined by analyzing the DNA in patients' tumors. Such a cocktail will be formulated to attack the culprit genes causing a specific variant.

This is the future; but today, the war on cancer remains a grueling battle of attrition.

John Mendelsohn, M.D.

Sixty-six years old—Houston, Texas
President of the University of Texas, M.D. Anderson Cancer Center

Life is terminal. But with cancer, we like to use the word incurable rather than terminal. Even though cancer is incurable, there are many patients who, with the medications we have, along with good luck and support from the good Lord, end up living five or even ten years with cancer; living *with* cancer, not getting rid of it. Unfortunately, for some patients, the end comes much earlier.

Our job as physicians is to keep up hope, pull every treatment alternative out of the box, and offer experimental therapies. Innovative new therapies are coming along, and they need to be tried. And the patient with the right attitude, who wants to participate, now has more and more choices.

Many times, experimental therapies don't work that well, while in other cases they do. That would be the hope. They're giving themselves a chance. And they're also helping the future, either ruling in or ruling out which experimental therapies should be further pursued and which, unfortunately, have to be discarded. There's still a lot left you can try, even if you've decided that the disease, using current technology, is incurable.

I know of one patient with chronic leukemia who came to M.D. Anderson in the 1980s and received standard therapy with a drug called Busulfan, which usually works for a few years. But, in this case, it failed, and she was expected to die soon. Then along came Interferon therapy, which we pioneered, and for which she volunteered to be a research subject. Interferon therapy controlled her disease for about five years, and then it started becoming resistant to Interferon.

A third new treatment came to our attention from China. This same patient volunteered to try it, and that worked for two or three years, but then it, too, failed, and the disease continued to progress. Next, there was a drug called Gleevec, which displayed miraculous activity against chronic myelocytic leukemia.

Today, her disease is in complete remission and she might possibly be cured. In the 1980s, when she was diagnosed with this disease, her life expectancy was three years, which is why this one, and hundreds more are the success stories I wish I could share with thousands of patients because they're the answer to the hope every patient has.

While we're always getting closer to a cure for cancer, realistically we're always further away than we want to be. When I was a kid, about 30 percent of cancers were curable. Now, about 60 percent are curable. Are we making progress? You bet. But our population's aging.

Even though the chance of dying from cancer has decreased, because there are so many older people, the total number of cancer patients has increased. And, now, as baby boomers hit their sixties and seventies, often living into their eighties, we're going to see a lot more cancer.

"We need to really let people know what cancer is. We need to give people the information they need in a language they can understand."

— *Scott Hamilton—testicular cancer,*
Olympic gold medalist figure skater

Patrick C. Walsh, M.D.

Sixty-three years old—Baltimore, Maryland
Director of the Brady Urological Institute at
The Johns Hopkins Medical Institutions

DNA is short for deoxyribonucleic acid. It is our genetic blueprint, and it's in every cell in our bodies. It's a chemical Morse code. It's the alphabet that our body uses to create every tissue, every protein, every enzyme, everything in our body. That alphabet spells out certain proteins. If the alphabet is damaged, there are misspellings; cells are misspelled, creating an environment where certain proteins are not made.

There are proteins called tumor-suppresser genes. These are checkpoint genes that are normally there to suppress tumors from developing. If they get damaged, they're not there to prevent cancer from forming. There are other genes called oncogenes. They're growth factors. If they get damaged, it's like stepping on the gas pedal; it makes the tumor grow faster. In addition, there are mismatched repair genes that repair damaged DNA. These are quality control genes, and if one or more of these inspector genes is muted, wide-spread mutations can occur, with disastrous results.

Cancer research is moving forward. I mean, we can always do better, but we're doing a lot better now than ten years ago. An American boy born today has a 16 percent risk of developing prostate cancer, and nearly a 3 percent risk of dying from it. However, we expect these numbers to improve. While I don't have a crystal ball, everyone is working extremely hard. In almost every other field of medicine, tremendous breakthroughs have occurred through antibiotics, immunizations, and all forms of treatment. I'm expecting there will be a cascade of discovery in the field of cancer.

Paul A. Marks, M.D.

Seventy-six years old—New York, New York
President Emeritus of Memorial Sloan-Kettering Cancer Center and
Member, Sloan-Kettering Institute for Cancer Research

I have a sense that we are moving at an accelerated rate toward new para-digms of cancer treatment, some of which seem very, very interesting. There are several approaches to therapy that are not based on a specific defect in a specific cancer, but rather they target a defect common to many cancers. That's pretty exciting.

We are involved in the development of small molecules that target enzymes called histone deacetylases, which are important regulators of gene expression. It turns out that when you inhibit them, you get a re-expression of genes that have been suppressed in cancer cells, and associated with this re-expression is a block in cell proliferation. These are relatively non-toxic agents.

This will be a new paradigm. We will have orally administered pills, and the most promising aspect of these agents is that they work on metastatic (spreading) cancer, which now has limited effective agents to treat it. Although there are a few instances where specific antibodies are effective in certain selective diseases, on the whole, metastatic cancer remains a very difficult disease to treat.

Cancer research is definitely focusing on interesting targets. As we come to understand the structure of these targets, we are able to make molecules that look like they are increasingly effective as anti-cancer agents and also possess acceptable tolerated side effects. In addition, it seems that the same pill can be used for many different cancers. While different cancers have different defects in the DNA, many cancers have certain defects in com-mon. These drugs will not cure the underlying cause of cancer, but they will arrest the growth of the cancer.

Therefore, when you succeed, what you are doing is turning cancer into a chronic disease (one you can live with), which isn't a bad result, partic-ularly if it doesn't interfere with your lifestyle.

Peter K. Vogt, Ph.D.

Seventy-one years old—La Jolla, California
Head, Division of Oncovirology and Professor, Department of Molecular and
Experimental Medicine at The Scripps Research Institute

A lot of headway is being made in cancer research and it is all in the area of the new targets emerging from the analysis of genetic changes in cancer cells. This means we can expect spectacular progress in specific genetically defined cancers very soon. A good example is chronic myelogenous leukemia.

Cancer is not one disease but hundreds of different diseases. They are all defined by tissue of origin, by genetic changes, and by the targets they represent. Some of the targets that have appeared come in relatively small niches of cancer. There are also other types of leukemia than the one I mentioned that are equally vulnerable and where we will probably see equal improvement in the near future.

I also think we will see a lot of rapid progress in fighting other types of cancers where genetic changes are being defined and where molecular targets appear that can be attacked by drugs. I am very confident that the whole landscape of cancer research and cancer treatment is about to change dramatically. We will have very specific drugs for very specific cancers.

In the future, we will be able to say at initial diagnosis that this patient has these and these and these genetic changes and hence, this is the appropriate cocktail of drugs that we have to apply. This is right around the corner.

Eventually, we will be able to say that every patient has his or her individual cancer. We will know enough about genetic changes and molecular changes to make these distinctions.

Anne Wallace, M.D., F.A.C.S.

Forty-one years of age—La Jolla, California
Director of the Breast Care Unit; surgical oncologist and plastic surgeon,
UCSD's Moores Cancer Center

We saw the first reduction in breast cancer in the 1990s, which was probably the result of better therapy. In the 21st century, headway is being made in understanding the molecular level of cancer in general, and understanding how various proteins and genes are expressed and how to better intercept that process.

This is still in its infancy, but I think it is really going to explode in the near future. This discovery will effect breast cancer treatment at the biologic level and will replace the kind of "slash and burn" treatment of chemotherapy and radiation.

The mammogram is now the best tool we have for early detection of breast cancer. We are moving toward digital mammography, which will be a great improvement. However, it is horribly expensive to use and therefore, it won't be readily available.

We have been reading articles in the newspapers the last couple of years saying that mammograms don't save lives. It's not because they don't do a really good job of finding cancer; it's because the cancer detected by mammograms is the type that probably wouldn't kill anyone. What we really need to do is figure out which cancers we are finding are biologically important. This is crucial to understand because a person thinks, If it's found early, I'm going to live. This is not necessarily the case. With respect to breast cancer, bigger is not always worse.

We don't need better mammograms; we need different mammograms. One thing we do have is MRIs. They are not a screening test for everyone, but for high risk women or women who have a different type of symptom, MRIs can be fabulous. It's not a replacement for mammograms, it's a supplement. It can see things a mammogram can't and mammograms can see things that MRIs can't. Imaging and imaging agents are definitely the keys to the future.

E. David Crawford, M.D.

Fifty-five years old—Denver, Colorado
Section Head of Urologic Oncology at the University of Colorado Health
Science Center and Chairman of the Prostate Cancer Education Council

Back in the late 1980s, most of the cases of prostate cancer that we found were not localized; they were advanced and incurable. That's because we didn't have early detection efforts. We didn't have public knowledge about prostate glands, nor did we even know what they were. We didn't have PSA (prostate-specific antigen) tests.

I did a lot of work with advanced prostate cancer and new treatments, so I saw people from all over the country. One of the men I treated was from Las Vegas. His name was Perry Lieber, and he was Howard Hughes' director of operations. Perry was in his eighties when he had prostate cancer and he had advanced disease, so I took care of him.

He asked me, "Why is it that this disease is always advanced when it's detected?" I said, "We just don't have enough people come in and get checked for it, just the rectal exam." Remember that this was before PSA tests, and Perry, being in public relations, said, "We've got to do something about that. We need a national campaign to raise awareness about prostate cancer and to promote early detection."

We talked about it, and we were going to launch it in Colorado and Nevada. Unfortunately, Perry died, but his widow was still very interested in the program and helped us out with some seed money. In 1989, we started Prostate Cancer Awareness Week in the United States. At that time, it was difficult to even get anybody to talk about it. Men were pretty quiet about their diseases. Bob Hope had prostate cancer, but he wouldn't talk about it. We finally got Rocky Bleier, the running back for the Pittsburgh Steelers, to do it because his grandfather had prostate cancer. He was great.

To launch Prostate Cancer Awareness Week, we did a little campaign that began with a press conference in New York. That year we got 10,000 men to come in from around the country. The next year it was 150,000; a year later it was 500,000; and it's been a million plus ever since.

Rudy Guiliani helped us. He did a public service announcement that was broadcast all over the country. We had the NFL as one of our supporters, and they created awareness at a number of their games and on their Web site. This year was probably our most successful. We are very interested in promoting awareness among African Americans because they have a high incidence of prostate cancer. This year we doubled the number of African Americans being screened.

We have learned a lot about screening, early detection, desired PSA levels, and new forms of PSA—free PSA, complex PSA. We are most excited about complex PSA. PSA exists in your blood in two forms. It exists in a free form, which is a PSA molecule; it also consists of PSA bound to protein, called complex PSA. When we originally measured total PSA with the tests, we measured both free and bound; but now we're finding that the bound PSA is a more specific way to detect prostate cancer. So, basically, we can still detect as many cases, but we can cut down on the number of biopsies that are done.

What we can say is that men who are screened on a yearly basis don't develop advanced prostate cancer because we catch it early. We've seen a rapid shift in the number of men with advanced disease. We've also seen some improvement in the survival rate, which we'd like to attribute to screening.

One of the papers I presented this spring at a couple of national meetings concerned the levels of PSA in relationship to relative risk of developing prostate cancer. This was from a large trial I was involved in, to look for screening for prostate, lung, colorectal (colon and rectum), and ovarian cancer. We found that of the men who had a PSA of less than one on their initial screen, only about 1 percent of them will develop an abnormality in five years. An abnormality means a PSA greater than four. This gives them a certain amount of assurance that they're okay. It also saves the healthcare industry half a billion to a billion dollars a year by eliminating unnecessary testing.

"As you get older, your genetic disposition becomes more prominent. This is particularly true if there is a family history of cancer. As doctors, we've looked at the illness side of genetics. I also believe there is a strong genetic side to the survivors of cancer."

— *Peder Shea, M.D., F.A.C.P.,*
F.A.C.C., Cardiovascular Diseases

Stephen H. Friend, M.D., Ph.D.

Forty-nine years old—West Point, Pennsylvania
President, Rosetta Inpharmatics, Inc.; Vice President, Basic Research,
Merck Research Laboratories, Merck & Co., Inc.

The thing that thrilled the clinician scientists in the mid-1980s was the identification of the genes called cancer genes, oncogenes, and tumor-suppresser genes. We'd get one and it would go on the front page of *The New York Times*, and everyone would be all excited. To put it in perspective, that's coming up on twenty years ago.

We now realize the complexity of cancer means the solution is not going to be one-size-fits-all for patients. Cancer is a series of diseases, a whole collection that has, unfortunately, been grouped together. We used to think all cancer was cancer. We now know that not all prostate cancer is prostate cancer, and not all breast cancer is breast cancer. The information we now have about how you treat a tumor is at the stage when history tells us that more selective therapies will soon be coming along.

The problem is that every time there is a small advance, it gets highlighted in such a way that it sounds like everything has been solved. It's the "cry-wolf phenomenon." Realistically, scientists have no idea when they'll have all the answers.

The pharmaceutical companies are now shifting from the absurd goal of finding a compound that will treat all patients to actually trying to find situations where a smaller set of patients can be very effectively treated. The Novartis compound Gleevec is an example of that. The goal is molecular targets as opposed to the old approach of putting the most toxic things you can think of into people, hoping that the tumor cells are weak, and that you can kill the tumor a little faster than you can kill the patient.

Some patients say the stronger the medicine and the worse the effect on them, the better they feel about their battle with cancer. That just isn't right. I compare that to the treatment of syphilis back in the 1920s. They would give patients infections to induce fevers and then feed them arsenic. That just doesn't make much sense to me. But at that time, it made sense to everyone. I'm hoping we're going to come out of the medieval concept that the harder on the patient the drug is, the more likely it will work to treat cancer.

I think that molecular targets, where you go in and selectively find something that is altered in the tumor that is not present in the normal cells, something that would selectively kill a tumor cell over a normal cell, is the direction our therapies have to go if we're going to find cures and achieve something other than just partial remissions.

When people ask, "Are we close to curing cancer?" I think anyone who tells you it's sooner than five years is unrealistic. I may be an optimist, but I think the time frame is just that, five years. So cancer survivors need to stay alive for five more years.

Right now the terrible thing is that there's too much hype out there. It creates a nation of numb readers. After they've heard this hype enough times it all becomes *The National Enquirer*. That's the saddest thing to me.

"New gene-profiling technology—the most innovative scientific technology available—allows us to view thousands of genes on a tiny DNA chip. By studying these gene profiles, we can zero in on those genes classified as problematic, indicating that a mutation in the gene could cause cancer in the cell.

"Another aggressive initiative we are undertaking is the Kinase Project, with the objective of identifying 'targeted therapies:' drugs that attack malignant cells and leave healthy cell unscathed."

— *Dr. Edward J. Benz Jr.,*
President, Dana-Farber Cancer
Institute, Boston Massachusetts

Andrew von Eschenbach, M.D.

Sixty-two years old—Bethesda, Maryland
Director of the National Cancer Institute

Cancer occurs when the genetic program in a cell goes haywire and the cell no longer obeys the rules of controlled growth and function. We know there are many kinds of cancers, that cancers have different manifestations, and that we need to take into account the complexity of cancer. You can't make blanket statements about cancer and expect them to apply universally.

You can't even make blanket statements about specific kinds of cancers. Our research is now telling us that even when we have forms of lymphoma that look exactly the same under the microscope, when we probe them from a genetic perspective, they are completely different and will behave completely differently to different therapies.

We are at a moment when the huge investment in research that began in 1971 with President Nixon's war on cancer, is beginning to pay dividends. That investment has helped us understand the disease. In 1971, we didn't.

The next challenge is not to just gather information, but to integrate it into the clinics. All this new knowledge is opening doors for us to be able to intervene in ways we never could before.

If the model of 20th century cancer care was to find the cancer and kill it, then we're going to take this new knowledge to do something different. For instance, as a urologic oncologist, the main operation I performed for prostate cancer was a radical prostectomy, which was introduced in this country in 1904. What urologists are now trying to do is understand the cancer, and based on that understanding, apply a discreet intervention to manipulate the cancer—retard it, reverse it, or prevent it.

"Within our lifetime, one of every two men will develop some form of cancer, and one of three females will do the same."

— Dr. Andrew von Eschenbach,
Director of the National Cancer
Institute

"Americans are eating themselves to death. A sixteen-year study, involving more than one million volunteers, by the American Cancer Society has concluded that an estimated 90,000 Americans die each year of cancer caused primarily by obesity. That makes obesity second only to smoking as a preventable cause of cancer."

— The New England Journal of Medicine

"It is simple to stop cancer before it starts. Just look at tobacco."

— Dr. Peter K. Vogt,
Professor, The Scripps Research
Institute (Smoking causes about
170,000 cancer deaths per year)

David Hodgens, M.D.

Fifty-eight years old—La Jolla, California
Medical Director of Radiation Oncology, Scripps Memorial Hospital

We are still fighting cancer with some of the same tools we've been using the last fifty to one hundred years. The main difference is that we are using more sophisticated techniques for such things as aiming radiation beams, directing chemotherapy drugs, and guiding cancer surgeons in the operating room. But mostly, we are using very similar tools to what we have been using for the past half-century, just in a more technical way.

The good news is that we are standing on the threshold of significant advances in our ability to actually target cancer cells as opposed to the normal tissues that are around them, which is one of the great difficulties that we have.

Cancer is as individual as each patient because cancer comes from the patient's own genetic material. This means that targeting cancer in an individual takes a unique approach for each person. Cancer cells may be similar in breast cancer patients and in prostate cancer patients because these cancers are similar to each other in terms of diagnosis. But the actual cancer cell in each individual breast cancer patient or prostate cancer patient may be a little different from another patient, and it takes individual targeting to overcome that difference.

Robert T. Abraham, Ph.D.

Fifty years old—La Jolla, California
Professor and Director, Program in Signal Transduction Research;
Director, Cancer Research Center, The Burnham Institute

Three decades have passed since President Nixon declared a war on cancer in America. The strategy was appropriately warlike – this most feared of human afflictions was to be brought to its knees by an overwhelming combination of scientific and clinical firepower, together with a dedicated infrastructure and superb technological resources.

As in all previous wars, the American taxpayers were asked to shoulder a substantial proportion of the costs associated with outfitting and maintaining this army of cancer researchers and medical doctors. The United States government funneled billions of dollars into academic institutions, private research foundations and clinics, and biotechnology companies, with the single-minded objective of ridding this country and the world of cancer.

My status report for the war on cancer is highly optimistic. To be sure, the enemy is still among us, shortening productive lives and causing untold suffering. And admittedly, we in the cancer research community have stumbled at times and raised false hopes at others. Nonetheless, cancer doctors at The Burnham Institute and other cancer centers around the country are now more excited than ever because we sense that a revolution in cancer prevention and treatment is already upon us.

Many years of painstaking labor have yielded a remarkably detailed picture of the cancer cell, and this knowledge is opening a Pandora's box of rational therapeutic approaches to attack this disease at its weakest points. Moreover, a remarkable feature of cancer research (and one reason that many scientists find the disease so endlessly fascinating) is that it reaches far beyond the boundaries of cancer itself. The war on cancer has yielded invaluable insights into the root causes and therapeutic management of seemingly unrelated diseases, such as rheumatoid arthritis and Alzheimer's disease.

The benefits of this nation's investment in cancer research are aptly compared to those stemming from our space exploration program. Not everyone agrees that our country should be spending large sums of money on space stations and the like, but the advances in computer, communications, and military technology made possible by our space program have touched virtually every corner of our society.

So, too, it goes for cancer research because when you get down to the nitty-gritty details, a cancer cell is nothing more than a normal body cell gone bad. In studying cancer cells, we cannot help but learn more about how healthy cells and tissues function and how they become involved in other disease processes, such as the chronic joint inflammation that plagues patients with arthritis.

At the war on cancer's inception, the general assumption was that we were tackling a single disease, regardless of the tissue of origin (e.g., breast, lung, or prostate). Of course, the first hard lesson from the field was that the enemy had many faces, and in spite of the occasional newspaper headline, most cancer researchers and clinicians quickly recognized that the development of a "magic bullet" cure for all types of cancer was an unrealistic goal.

However, this somewhat sobering reality is more than counterbalanced by a greater reality; that is, three decades of dedicated work have yielded an incredibly detailed view of the process by which normal cells are transformed into "rogue cells" that play by their own rules and build their own tissues (i.e., tumors) in inappropriate locations in the body, to the detriment of the human host.

In earlier days, cancer was diagnosed primarily by the pathologist, who scanned biopsy specimens for signs of the deranged cell and tissue architecture characteristic of an established tumor. Unfortunately, by the time an observable mass was found in such a biopsy, the disease had already spread to other sites (metastasized), which meant that the chances that surgery, chemotherapy, or other treatments would lead to long-term survival, were very slim. Furthermore, the most popular treatments of the day were severe poisons in and of themselves – the hope being that the drugs would kill the tumor before they killed the patient.

We now conceptualize cancer in radically different terms. We have in hand a detailed view of cancer at the molecular level, and we have defined a set of abnormalities that largely account for the abnormal and potentially deadly behavior of all human cancer cells. Collectively, these abnormalities allow cancer cells and the tumor masses that they form to ignore the boundaries that limit normal cell and tissue growth.

The complexity of this disease arises from the fact that developing tumors can take many different paths to achieve the endpoint of unrestricted growth; the paths taken for any individual tumor are usually quite different from those followed by another tumor. The clinical ramifications of these findings are profound. For example, we now recognize that even visually similar breast tumors from different patients often show a high level of heterogeneity at the molecular level. These molecular differences will translate into critical differences in tumor aggressiveness and responsiveness to therapy. Moreover, the identification of pathways that become deregulated during tumor development brings into focus specific weaknesses that can be attacked to therapeutic advantage.

In laboratory jargon, we term these chinks in the disease armor as "targets," and new targets for anticancer drug discovery are now moving through the research pipeline at a dizzying pace. The sequencing of the human genome, which was funded in part through our own National Institutes of Health, has truly moved the target identification process into warp speed.

As of this writing, new-age weaponry of every sort – proteins, antibodies, and chemicals – is making its way through the gauntlet of clinical cancer trials. Within the next one to two decades, we predict that most cancer patients will be treated on an individualized basis, with the particular cocktail of new-age drugs tailored to the specific sets of molecular abnormalities present in their tumors. Side effects will be dramatically reduced, quality of life increased, and the word "cure" will become much more commonplace in our cancer clinics.

We have new challenges to be sure, not the least of which is identifying that population of cancer patients most likely to benefit from this new generation of molecularly targeted drugs. However, we have come so far during the past three decades that the remaining obstacles appear to be mere speed bumps on the road to a cure for many types of cancer.

This book documents the perseverance and bravery of cancer survivors. Our goal as cancer researchers and clinicians is to ensure that many more of today's cancer patients will be casting themselves as tomorrow's long-term survivors. We look forward to hearing their stories of bravery and perseverance as well.

"Cancer survivors have to live with the fact that there is now no cure for cancer. You're in remission, never cured. There's always the chance of cancer returning and metastasizing (spreading) to some other part of your body. Sometimes the second time around is not as traumatic as the first because you know what to expect. On the other hand, sometimes it is more traumatic because you know what to expect."

— *Charlie Jones—prostate cancer,*
co-author

Chapter Two
Coping with Cancer

Perhaps the coping aspect of cancer should have its own personal DNA because each of us has an individual approach, and the process of coping has many different phases.

First, one has to cope with the diagnosis—yes, I have cancer. That realization is immediately followed by numerous questions, the foremost being, "Why me?" and "Will I die from this cancer?" These are followed by, "What now?" and later down the road, "Now that my treatment is over, what's next?"

There are many ways to cope with cancer, and as you will see, the path you take is entirely up to you.

"This is something personal. I flew missions in North Vietnam, parachuting in over enemy lines, but nothing was as scary as having my doctor look me in the eye and say, 'You've got cancer.' Cancer is bipartisan. It attacks anybody and anything."

— *Randy "Duke" Cunningham—prostate cancer, U.S. congressman, Republican, California*

John Mendelsohn, M.D.
Sixty-six years old—Houston, Texas
President of the University of Texas, M.D. Anderson Cancer Center

First of all, when a patient is told they have cancer, they've lost control. Everyone feels they have some control over what they do, over their daily activities, but then all of a sudden, there's no control. It's replaced by an incredible uncertainty.

Secondly, they're forced to put themselves in an area of trust that's new, with someone they've, usually, never met before. This is a very jolting experience. It's a very difficult challenge to realize that, as wise as doctors are and as much as medicine has accomplished, you cannot have rationally perfect answers to the question of what are the best steps in therapy for you to take. There're going to be unknown variables. Doctors can explain risks and statistics, but they can make no guarantees.

The third area is the problem of how to plan for the future. We're all very busy. We all have schedules stuck to our refrigerator door. Every minute is accounted for and then, all of a sudden, how can I take that trip if I've got to do my chemo? What's going to happen six months from now? What happens if my cancer recurs; they say there's a 50 percent chance of recurrence? You have to recalibrate your whole life, in terms of how to plan, down to the minute. That's a tremendous challenge.

The coping has to be done by the patient and by his or her support system. The doctor becomes an important part of that support system. That's one of the rewarding things about being a specialist in cancer; you are not only providing special expertise and skills in treating a disease, but you're also providing experience and skills in caring for the patient.

At M.D. Anderson, we always talk about the difference in the synergy in caring for the patient and treating the cancer. We emphasize caring for the patient's needs and drawing them out in those areas of control. We help the patient accept the fact that this can't all be rational, and we help them in trying to accept the uncertainties in planning the future.

It's amazing how quickly, if you are interested in the patient, you develop a trusting relationship, how quickly barriers go down, and how quickly you become a real confidante of the patient and have a chance to participate in their innermost concerns. And that's, perhaps, equally rewarding for a specialist in this area, along with the satisfaction of applying scientifically proven therapies.

Every patient draws on his or her own personal experience to cope with cancer. There are some people who depend on their religion and the affiliations they have in their church. Other people are more, shall we say, new-age in their approach and are into mind-expanding procedures and yoga and the wisdom that can be brought from other cultures. There are courses and advisors in all these areas.

At M.D. Anderson, we have a small area called A PLACE OF WELLNESS (and there are three dots after wellness, so it's A PLACE OF WELLNESS . . .) where patients can sit down and talk with someone about alternative ways of finding support and learn what resources are available in Houston. We will send people to the youth center, we will send them to yoga classes, we will send them to art classes, and we will send them to meditation classes.

Some of these services are provided by M.D. Anderson, and some are provided by other organizations in the community. We encourage patients to try any alternative that strengthens their fight against cancer. It's important for patients to accept what is happening to them, and at the same time, to maintain their exercise and nutrition programs. Having a sense of control can also lift their spirits.

"I tell new cancer patients: Don't fight it. You have to accept it. Ask the questions you want the answers to. Make sure your doctor is someone you are extremely comfortable with. Decide within yourself the type and size of personal support system you want and need. Maintain a good attitude, and don't forget you are going to be more tired than you'll think you'll be. That's just the way it works."

— *Ellie Glaser—cancer of the lymph nodes,*
working single parent

Maryann Rosenthal, Ph.D.

Fifty-four years old—La Jolla, California
Licensed clinical and consulting psychologist

There are five steps in coping with cancer. They are denial, anger, bargaining, depression and, finally, acceptance. You have to move through each step to get to the acceptance stage.

First, there's the denial, "Why me?" Or "It can't be me." Or "They're going to find something else." You have to let people sit with that for a while. They need support and then they move on.

If they don't go into the next step, anger, I help them get there. It's important to be a little bit angry. "I'm pissed off I have cancer. Why doesn't he have cancer? I've always taken care of myself. My brother smokes and I've never smoked. It's not fair." You don't want to remain in any of the steps for very long, but you have to go through all of them.

The next step, bargaining, brings in prayer life or spirituality, without which I don't think anybody can get through this disease. I always ask, "What's your spiritual life like?" That's a real key for me as to what direction I try to take them. I'm not going to give them spirituality but if they have it, it's always going to make the journey a lot easier.

Then there's depression. I'm always looking for that. It can come from the medication, the radiation, the chemo, and also from fatigue. That's when I try to keep them as adaptive as possible, by getting them as involved as possible in their life.

The final step is acceptance and with that, comes hope and quality of life. I have to get them to this stage because if they're trapped, they're not going to be happy.

There are people who don't have any support, and I do everything I can to help them get a support system, even if it's an animal that they love. I try to get them involved. Sometimes I'm their only support, and that's hard for me because of therapeutic boundaries. The key is detachment without disconnection. If I didn't detach, if I got sucked into a patient's cancer, I wouldn't be able to help them. I have to be able to stay a bit detached, but not disconnected.

Therapists try different things. I try to meet the client where the client is at that time. Not where I want them to be, or where I think they should be, but where, after spending some time with them, they are. My job as a therapist is to bring that out and help them because sometimes, even they don't know where they are.

―――――――

"When you have one of those down days, wear something red. That will definitely brighten you up."

> — *Maryann Rosenthal, Ph.D.,*
> *licensed clinical and consulting*
> *psychologist*

―――――――

"Mentally, I know this sounds simple, but I've counted my blessings. There are so many people in this world who are worse off than I am. Also, I've counseled other people. It helps me to help others. I've learned how to quiet my mind and my body, and be able to go inward in meditation."

> — *Doris Ellsworth—non-Hodgkins*
> *lymphoma*

Don Ritt, M.D.
Sixty-seven years old—Rancho Santa Fe, California
Practicing gastroenterologist

A recent patient was a man in his seventies with pancreatic cancer. There is a very interesting technique by which you ultrasound the pancreas through an endoscope. Then you find your spot; you put a needle into it through the endoscope, right through the stomach and into the pancreas to get tissue out.

The first report was that it was not cancer, so there was a huge sense of relief. But a couple days later I had the task of telling him, "The first results were wrong. You actually do have cancer."

He stepped back and said, "Well, I'll just have to beat it." That was the way he faced all the problems in his life. He was a very successful and highly respected businessman. If he had a problem, he'd just take a deep breath, go at it, and handle it.

He went through his chemotherapy very nicely. He maintained a positive attitude. But as he started to deteriorate, he was quite clear in his statements, "I don't want to push on very much more." And, "Whatever happens, happens. Make sure I get my pain taken care of pretty well." Which is what we did.

He died about a year or so after the diagnosis was made. His first reaction was, "This is just another problem and I'll take care of it." He coped with that the same way he coped with every other problem.

Some of the religious backgrounds of individual patients are important. I have a young man who is in his late thirties. He has all sorts of colitis and then he developed colon cancer, which is not horribly unusual in that setting. He has widespread metastasis, and we're very worried about him.

However, he has enormous religious faith, and the minister from his church spends time with him. He's just fine. He believes God is going to save him and he's done nicely with his chemo and radiation. We can't see any tumor now on the CT scan. He's a long way from being out of the woods, but his approach is that he's fine. It doesn't matter; he's already talked to God, and God is going to take care of it. He has his entire church praying for him. Everyone is very upbeat, convinced that God will save him. So his method of coping is to become completely immersed in a religious approach. It seems to be working.

"I've decided not to suffer through my experimental treatments because I want quality of life. I hope and pray I have thirty years left, but I know I'm going to enjoy whatever time I have. God is the ultimate healer, and it's God's choice. I'm at peace with that."

> — *Vicki Schmidt—glioblastoma,*
> *mother of San Francisco Giant pitcher*
> *Jason Schmidt*

John Trombold, M.D., F.A.C.P.

Sixty-seven years old—La Jolla, California
Medical Director of the Scripps Stevens Cancer Center

I've always been fascinated with seeing how some patients handle adversity compared to others. I've always felt, but never been able to prove, that we all have our own coping mechanism that kicks in when we face a traumatic situation. Having cancer certainly fits that category.

I also believe that this coping mechanism has been programmed by our parents. I used to see internal medicine patients, and I remember one man who came into my office and said, "I have the flu and I want a penicillin shot." "Hold it," I said, "I'm the doctor, and after an examination I'll decide what medication you should have." As I was looking him over, I added, "By the way, when you were a kid, what did your father do when he caught the flu?" My patient replied, "He always got a shot of penicillin."

I think it's an extension of how you cope with whatever you've been coping with before. I used to argue with social workers and psychologists. They'd say, "No, we can counsel these people, and they'll cope a lot better than they did before."

I don't agree. I think the coping mechanism you have going into cancer is the same coping mechanism you'll have when you get there.

For some people, everything is a major issue. Some of the people who I think are most stressed are the ones who can't separate the major items from the minor items on a daily basis. They're uptight all the time because they want to get all these things done in one day, but they can't.

There's an old adage about what makes one feel really good. It's all about starting something, no matter what, and finishing it. It may be a crossword puzzle. If you complete it, you've had a good day. If you're tired from cancer and from your treatment, then just start something simple and try to finish it. If that's all you get to that day, then that's all you can do.

"Some people cope really well and some cope terribly. The question is, can you change when you're forty-five or fifty or fifty-five? I think your fiber's pretty well set by then. And I'm pretty damn sure at seventy you're not going to change hardly at all. It would take another Pearl Harbor."

— *Dr. John Trombold*

"I have several cancer patients who, after they have completed their treatment, have gone on-line with cancer buddies throughout the world. They meet Internet friends who have had the same cancer treatment and are in the same state of recovery."

— *Dr. John Trombold*

Joel Bernstein, M.D., F.A.C.P.
Forty-eight years old—La Jolla, California
Board certified medical oncology

I have patients who hate the treatments for Hodgkin's lymphoma, which is treatable. Then, a few weeks after their treatment is over, they hit their panic button, which screams, "What do I do now to keep the cancer away?" I tell them, "You've already done it. You don't need that crutch anymore."

Another type of patient is the young man with testicular cancer. After going through a very difficult treatment, this patient suddenly becomes a weight lifter. It's a male thing, a reaction to being traumatized by treatment. He immediately loses twenty pounds of fat and puts on twenty pounds of muscle. When you see someone do this, it's really quite something.

One of my testicular cancer patients was upset that his time on his stationary bike was a little off. This was a patient who had replaced a third of his blood volume. He should have been sleeping it off in bed, not getting on a bicycle and cranking for an hour and a half.

We really don't know all the things that radiation does. There are all these chemical analyses of what goes on, but they're an inadequate explanation of what patients feel and experience. It's as though your body has been inflamed. Just imagine a block of tissue on the inside of your body having a sunburn.

It really saps your strength so that coping with that inflammation can be exhausting. For you to heal, you have to build protein, and that takes time. Your body's restorative program is on hold until that injury has recovered.

When patients tell me they're feeling great, that's great! When they tell me they feel lousy, I say, "Then choose another day to feel great." There are different ways of coping.

"In an odd way, having cancer was easier than recovery—at least in chemo I was doing something, instead of just waiting for it to come back."

— *Lance Armstrong—cancer of the testicle, lungs, abdomen, and brain, he recovered and went on to win the world's most grueling test of human endurance, the Tour de France, in 1999, 2000, 2001, and 2002*

Wendy Lythgoe—Hodgkins lymphoma
Twenty-seven years old—Seattle, Washington
Downhill skier

I was actually fighting my body for about three years with rheumatoid arthritis. I thought that's all I was dealing with at that time. I lived in Seattle and the weather there really affected me. So I decided to move to Southern California about two years ago. A few weeks later, I went into the hospital with a swollen leg. I thought it was because I had previously broken it while ski racing in Alaska. I love the downhill. I love the speed. I was fearless.

I assumed the swelling had something to do with the rod and screws in my leg. I was already dealing with arthritis, and I didn't think it could get much worse than that. They checked me into the hospital for five days and did a biopsy. Next, they took out a lymph node, and then it got worse, they told me it was cancer, Hodgkin's lymphoma.

I now believe that the rheumatoid arthritis came out of my body trying to fight the cancer. I'd gone to all the right specialists in Seattle. It just wasn't found. I think the most frustrating part was that I had been fighting my body and meanwhile everyone was saying I was all right. So, finally, I got to the right doctor, Dr. Joel Bernstein, who set me on the right path.

I went through three months of chemotherapy and a month of radiation, and I'm in the clear now. I feel so good, and my arthritis is under control. It was a really scary time. It was almost surreal. I couldn't believe that I had been fighting my body for so long, and there was a solution for it.

However, I'm having a more difficult time now coping with it than I did when I went through the chemotherapy. It was a scare and shock at first. Right now I'm in the clear, but I'm finding that I'm more depressed than I ever have been through the entire procedure.

I honestly think that the cancer was like the straw that broke the camel's back with me. Even though I had gone through so much in the last seven years I said, "I can still fight this battle." And I fought it, but now I'm really tired, just exhausted. I'm tired of fighting. I'm tired of fighting my body. Rheumatoid arthritis is so painful. There was a period of six months where I couldn't put on my socks because I couldn't move my hands.

I don't think negatively, but right now it's like I don't even know who I am. I'm finding out all over again. I don't know the answers. I think it's to be honest with myself, and with everyone around me. This is how I feel, I don't know why. I have very supportive and loving family and friends.

I don't think it's how far you fall, it's how far you bounce back. My bounce is just a little shallow right now. I'm kind of deflated. I'm trying to put the air back in the ball.

Ultimately, I know I'll get through it, but right now I walk with a heavy heart, and I'm not quite ready to turn corners in my life again.

"There's a possibility my acute/promyelocyte leukemia can come back, and that's always a thought that crosses my mind. I don't know if there was a specific moment when I felt I had won; it was just a long, arduous battle."

— *Corina Morariu—leukemia,*
world's number one ranked women's
tennis doubles player in year 2000,
now making a comeback after a
two-year battle with cancer

James Sherrill, Jr. M.D., F.A.C.S.—colon cancer, prostate cancer
Sixty-seven years old—La Jolla, California
Diplomate, American Board of Ophthalmology

Colon cancer comes in three stages: A, B, and C, and as they go down the alphabet, they get worse. I had a C, and in 1980, life expectancy at that time was about two years. So why am I alive? I decided to change my life— the way I practiced, how I dealt with stress, my spirituality, my lifestyle, everything. At that time I was young. I hadn't been in practice a long time, and I had three little kids under the age of ten. There were a lot of buzz words I learned in this business, but denial is not a river. There are some things you need to do and know, and accept and change.

The most important aspect is your spiritual life because that determines how you deal with your problems. When I got prostate cancer five years ago, because of the support groups I'd been with every week for over eighteen years because of my colon cancer, it didn't even make a blimp on the radar screen. It was a nothing.

In our support groups we talk about good cancers, bad cancers. We talk about the gift of cancer, and we talk about how to handle it. The way you handle it is the answer to the question, how's your spiritual life? The way you answer that is how you are going to do 99.99 percent of the time. Now I'm not suggesting you go out and become a foot-washing Catholic or Baptist, but I am saying, "Life is in the state of mind."

One of the problems men have is that we don't share intimacies, we share experiences. Women share intimacies. Women nurture, women support. Men, in general, cannot communicate on a gut level because of testosterone and the way we're brought up. Cancer brings about a whole middle life changing process. Remember, "Life is in the state of mind." Your mind and how you treat it, is going to dictate how you do.

You need to change, you've got to get rid of the stress. Every study shows that stress, malignant disease, and life are all correlated. If you have heavy stress, you do poorly; if you have no stress, you do well. The life survival of people who get rid of their stress and change they're *modus operundi* far exceeds that of people who don't.

Cancer is a mental disease. You say to me, "Jim, you're full of it; it's a physical disease." But it's a part of life, and life is not a dress rehearsal. Life is in the state of mind. How your mind works is how you're going to work and how you're going to handle it.

When you get to the point where you say, "I have a great spiritual life," you are going to do great. There is a difference between a spiritual life and a religious life. I live with a lady who never goes to church, but her spiritual life is incredible. Me, I'm a guy who has to go to church. When I got colon cancer in 1980, I went back to church real fast. I'm not saying God saved me, but I am saying that his presence, and the lectures, meetings, reading, talking, and communing, all enabled my brain to handle my cancer.

Do you believe in God? Do you believe in a greater being? I don't care what you are: a Muslim, a Hindu, a Jew. It's about spirituality, the greater being up there. There is a saying, "Let go and let God." Turn it over to the Lord, let Him take care of it. It's a process that takes a long time. The way you do it is you sit down and talk to guys who have been there. You need to get your mind in a frame where you can say, "Let go and let God. I'm not in control here." Those are the phrases. You will learn them as you go along. You've got to turn it over to the Lord, whoever that Lord is, and say, "You know, I'm going to get rid of this stress, and here's how I'm going to do it." You exercise and you learn to relax. You're not in control, and that's the problem. We're all control freaks, at least most men are.

"There are some people who have very small tumors that you could cure with almost anything; you could probably hit them on the head. And there are some tumors that surgery or radiation doesn't even touch. But we're doing better."

> — Dr. Patrick Walsh,
> Professor of urology, The Johns Hopkins Medical Institutions

---

"In many areas there are cancer support programs where you can go and get encouragement and talk to people who are going through exactly what you are going through. One of the problems with this format, and I've checked them out, is that sometimes a person who is not doing very well dominates the program, and everybody becomes horribly depressed by the time they leave. So if you are going to try this, do some homework on the group first."

> — Dr. Gerald Wahman,
> Senior urologist, Sparks Medical Plaza

"If you take a calendar and mark your good days, at the end of the month you'll look back and see yourself having more good days than bad. Day by day, or week by week, you don't see it."

> — Dr. Richard Hall,
> Diplomate, American Board of Urology

Kurt Simpson

Thirty-seven years old—Westlake Village, California
Sales executive, talks about his father's lung cancer

My dad is sixty-eight now. He has always been extremely strong and extremely healthy. He's the type of guy who would not go to the doctor unless he was on his deathbed. I can count on one hand the number of times he's been to a physician since I was sixteen years old. He's not a complainer, just a very strong person. When he got sick, he'd be down one day and then back to work the next.

About two years ago, he wasn't feeling well. He started to loose his energy and got kind of sluggish. On New Year's Eve, he went into the hospital with pneumonia. When they did a chest x-ray, they found a huge, golf-ball size tumor in his left lung. They treated him for the pneumonia and ran some tests, along with doing some biopsies.

One day after he came home, they called and told him he had lung cancer. This was devastating news and he and my mom crawled into bed in the middle of the day and just laid there, crying for hours. The only time I'd ever seen my dad cry was when I was in the hospital with knee surgery and my knee was ripped open with all kinds of tubes coming out. To see my father cry was a pretty heavy thing. He was pretty torn up.

My dad is a self-made man, with barely a high school education, yet he built a multimillion-dollar company from scratch. Nothing ever stopped him, and he is the strongest man I have ever met. In my mind, he was my idol and everything that I ever wanted to be as a man. When I saw him break down and I watched the glimmer go out of his eyes that first week when he found out he had lung cancer, I thought, Oh my God, he's vulnerable, and not only is he vulnerable, is he going to survive?

We went through about two weeks where the walls in everybody's life just got knocked down. Then we found out he could have surgery. He basically said, "Here's what I have to do. I have to take a run at it and see if I can kick this thing." He had surgery, and they removed two-thirds of his lung. One of the bronchial airways was kinked in the one-third of the lung that was left, so he had a hard time even breathing.

He developed a staph infection in the hospital and they treated him with Vancomycin, which is one of the most powerful antibiotics known to man, to make sure they could cure him of the staph infection and pneumonia. It was touch and go for a while because of the surgery as well as the infection.

They had him on heavy doses of morphine, and he would literally see spots on the wall. He also thought aliens were harvesting his body parts, which he would tell me about in the middle of the night. (I slept right beside him in the hospital.) He'd wake up and say, "The walls are raining," or "They're coming to get my body parts."

To hear that from my father was probably one of the most traumatic things I'd ever gone through in my life. Here was a man with the mental fortitude of a steel tank, who doesn't get rattled at anything, and he was telling me that his organs were being harvested and all this other bizarre stuff. It was just a terrible scenario.

Once they pulled him off the morphine and switched him to other medication, the hallucinations started to go away, and they finally cured him of the staph infection and sent him home. It was a really long recovery process. He had a hard time breathing because this one little airway was kinked. He went to UCLA where they were going to try to put a stint in, but the stint wouldn't work in the area where his lung was tweaked. Then we had another scare: They thought they found a lump on his good lung. They took biopsies of his lymph nodes, his other lung, the old lung, and everything came out okay. So far so good.

However, from my dad's perspective, cancer never goes away. You never have 100 percent certainty that it's gone. In the back of your mind, you always have the knowledge that it is still in your body, so you're hypersensitive to every little ache and pain. You're convinced you still have cancer. With an appendix, you cut it out and you move on. With a heart problem, you put in a heart valve and you have a 70 percent chance of living and a life expectancy of ten years. But with cancer, you just don't know. Even if they technically say it's gone, you really don't know if it's gone or not. My dad says that's the part he struggles with most today, just not knowing whether or not the cancer is really gone.

I have also come to the realization that he's not going to be the same person that he was. Mentally or physically, he's not going to be able to do the same things. He has days where he's convinced he still has cancer. And he has days when he says, "You know what? It is what it is and I just have to immerse myself in my family, my work, or whatever I enjoy doing to keep my mind away from it." That's where he is today. My mom also has to manage her expectations that he is not going to be the same guy. He's going to have bad days, and he's going to have good days. That's just the way it is right now. That's what this disease has dealt our family, and we just have to find the best way to handle it.

Linda Merkins—breast cancer that metastasized to her bones, liver, and brain over a ten-year period
Fifty-eight years old—La Jolla, California
Wife, mother, and grandmother

I've coped really well. I just don't have cancer on the weekend. I don't have cancer on any holidays, and I don't have cancer in the evenings, generally speaking. I simply refuse to acknowledge it. By 5:00 P.M. on Friday, I'm done with cancer. I stop having cancer until Monday morning. It does amazing things for your psyche. It also allows your family to become normal, and you to become normal, and to think about normal stuff.

I have been very lucky, I don't get terribly sick. I get tired sometimes and, once in a while, I get queasy. I never lose weight. I just gain it. After ten years, cancer is just something that I have. I feel like it's never going to go away. With any luck at all, the technology will stay enough ahead of me to keep me alive. And so far it has. I mean, I'm having surgeries and drugs and stuff that weren't around ten years ago.

Really, denial is what I use. But I'm not stupid. I know that Monday through Friday I have to pay attention. I never miss a doctor's appointment. I never ignore it.

There's nothing you can do about cancer on the weekend. So why have it? Why bother with it? Generally speaking, I won't discuss it from Friday at 5:00 P.M. until Monday at 8:00 A.M.

The other way I cope is I have almost all my treatments in Texas, so I leave my cancer down there. That helps enormously, to just leave your cancer someplace else.

I know people who think the best thing that ever happened to them was cancer. They finally got the attention they needed from their children and from others. They've got something that makes them really special. I've never thought cancer is a really special thing to have. I think it is a real drag.

I don't spend any time feeling sorry for myself. About nine years ago, around the time of the recurrence of my cancer, my stepdaughter's mother was in a hideous automobile accident. She has been in a semi-comatose state for nine years. Lots worse things can happen to you than having cancer.

I don't have any kind of major philosophy. I don't have any kind of incredible story. It's just that I refuse to think about dying. I hate it when people say, "We're all going to die." My response to that is, "You first." I don't have time for that now. I don't have time to be sick. What I have time for is a lot of kids, a lot of grandchildren, and I want to see how it all turns out.

"If I'm starting to have one of those really bad days, I just remind myself that somewhere in the world it's 5:00 p.m."

— *Linda Merkins*

Vern Marshall, Sr.—pancreatic cancer

Sixty-seven years old—Portland, Oregon
Football official for forty-five years (thirteen as an NFL line judge)
His story is shared by his son, Vern Marshall, Jr., also a football official.

Dad was diagnosed with pancreatic cancer, which is one of the most deadly forms of cancer. And although it was taking its toll on his body, he was still set to referee a high school football game between Roosevelt and Madison.

On our way to the high school stadium, his cancer again took the upper hand, forcing me to stop the car so he could throw up. But he kept going, because he was on his way to do what he loved doing his entire life, officiate a football game. We had assigned a high school crew, and I was on it with three other local guys. But little did he know what was in store for him.

He hadn't been in the officials' dressing room that long, when the high school athletic director came in and said to the other high school officials, "Fellows, we need you for a few minutes. We need to move some cars." Then, just as they left, in walked his old crew chief in the NFL, Red Cashion. Red looked down at Dad and continued walking towards his locker. You should have seen the look on Dad's face when Red walked in. But Red didn't say a word; he just kept walking. Right behind him was Terry Gierke, another former NFL crewmate, and Jack Barger, a Pac-10 conference official for twenty-five years. Jack was followed by two more NFL buddies, John Alderton and Nate Jones. Suddenly, there was ninety-six years of NFL officiating experience in that room, preparing to work a game between two high schools with one victory between them.

I tell you, Dad lit up like a Christmas tree when those guys walked into the dressing room. It was just amazing. Red was great. He turned around and said, "We heard you could use a little help on this one." Dad looked back at him and said, "If we can't get it done with this crew, it can't get be done."

When we came out of the locker room, there was another surprise, more than 100 officials from Portland, Salem, and other areas, all in their black and white striped uniforms, lined the entrance to the field to greet Dad.

They applauded him every step of the way. You should have seen the look on his face; he had tears welling up. I was so proud of him.

Dad handled the coin toss and I ended up working as the umpire, something I'd never done in my life. I'd never been in there with the linebackers, I've always worked deep and outside, but I told him, "Dad, I'm going to be with you every step of the way."

I had so much anxiety because we had people coming in from all over, and I didn't know if Dad was going to feel good enough to work the game. But there he was, with a tube sticking out of his body and a pouch tucked under his uniform to collect fluids from the surgery he had the previous week.

Madison got the opening kickoff, took it down the length of the field and scored. Dad got his hands up over his head signaling touchdown, and then he came over to me and said, "Vern, I'm just so cold." I said, "No problem, Dad. We'll get you your long- sleeve jersey." We got him his jersey, and I knew that once he got off to the sideline, my brother Joe would wrap him in a blanket and he'd be surrounded by good friends.

Then I slipped over to be the line judge, John Alderton went to umpire, and Red went to referee. We didn't skip a beat, it was just like clockwork. The way everything unfolded, you couldn't have written a better script. It was just amazing.

Dad has a great passion for officiating sports. He always said there is nothing better than officiating a football game on an autumn day where there's a warm breeze, the leaves are changing color, the sky is ocean blue without a cloud, and the warm sun is touching your shoulders. He says that he'll be smiling down on us, giving us a pat on the back, because there is nothing better than working with a good crew of officials.

Dad has a way with words, and he's got a heart of gold. He has so many good friends, and he's touched so many lives. Through sports, education, and everything he's done, he's lived a wealthy life, as far as friends are concerned.

Even though Dad had worked a Super Bowl, our dream was to work a high school game together, and we did.

Elizabeth Davidson—ovarian cancer, twice
Seventy-three years of age—Los Angeles, California
Wife and homemaker

When the doctor told me the first time that I had ovarian cancer, I couldn't believe it. I'm in very good health, and I've never been sick. I really didn't say, "Why me?" However, Marian, my sister, said, "Well, you know the divorce caused it. It was all that grief you went through." I do think stress had something to do with it. I also had a very stressful job at the music center.

The first time I was diagnosed, I said, "All right. This won't be a problem. I'll get over it." I always had faith that things would be okay. I was a little shaken when the cancer returned after a year and a half.

My first chemotherapy was Taxol, which is an absolute "hair fall out" chemotherapy. While I still had hair, I had been advised to go and get a wig as closely similar to my own hair as possible. My daughter Diana was visiting after I got out of the hospital, and she took me out to a wig place. I can remember hardly having the strength to sit on the stool while they went back to try and find something.

My hair did fall out. It came out in the shower by the handfuls. It was just awful. I had my wig there, so I think it's important to plan for the side effects that you know are going to happen. I had such a mixture of things, and everything affects you differently.

Some people tell me they feel better during chemo because they're fighting cancer. You're thinking that the chemo is destroying the tumors. It's such a clever disease, and it changes forms and gets used to one toxin while it survives others. It's very insidious.

I was in remission for about a year and a half. I was going in and having it monitored every three months. It has always been the medication that's made me so sick, not the cancer, which is fortunate. But you just can't let it have its way.

It's now been three years. I started in April, right after my seventieth birthday. So, it's been a long time. Some of the chemotherapy worked for awhile and then the numbers started going up again, so I've had maybe five or six different kinds. I just hope they don't run out of different things to try. But anyway, I don't dwell on it.

Every type of chemotherapy has different side effects. One even let my hair grow back in. Last summer we went up to Deer Valley and did some hiking. I took the chair lift up and walked down. It was a little more walking than I normally do. By the end of the week, my feet had started swelling so I couldn't get into any of my shoes. I had to go to an art fair and buy a pair of sandals so I could get home on the plane.

That was the end of the Taxol because the side effects negated the good it had done. But it was a very easy chemotherapy to take compared to what I'm having now, which is really chewing up my digestive system. It's called 5FU. It's Fluorouracil. It's the internal version of Effudex, which when put on your face, brings out the skin cancers, which peel off and eventually go away. The side effects are annoying, to say the least. It brings out stuff on your skin so you're itching all the time, have watery eyes, a dry mouth, and sores in the mouth.

As you know, medicine is not a science, it's an art. You never know; there are so many variables in the cancer itself. It's sort of like throwing things against the wall and seeing what sticks. You just can't think about it. You just have to endure it.

So many people have given me self-help books and things to read. I guess I'm just too much of a pragmatic person. I'd rather worry about whether or not I've fed my orchids. Everyone has his own method. I don't like to think about it a lot. I focus on living my normal life. Everyone copes in a different way, and my first rule of coping is to get out of bed.

Harold Shively, M.D., F.A.C.C., F.A.C.P.—melanoma
Sixty-five years of age—La Jolla, California
Cardiologist

I had a melanoma, which was a total surprise, although I've played baseball and lived outdoors a good part of my life. Like many men in Southern California now in their mid-sixties, I have spent a lot of time on beaches with my shirt off. I was getting ready to go play baseball in Arizona in the old men's league. I'm a pitcher for a team in men's Senior League hardball, and I'm throwing as hard as I ever did, the ball just doesn't go as fast. In college, I threw in the low nineties, now I throw in the low seventies.

During my check-up, my wife was there, and she said something was on my back. The dermatologist didn't really think much about it, but he snipped it off and sent it to pathology. When it came back, it was a melanoma, real thin, but the cells were lined up single file going down a hair root. You couldn't actually see the bottom of it.

The thickness of a melanoma has some prognostic implications. The problem is, when it travels down a hair follicle, you don't really know how thin it is or what to grade it. This one would've been four millimeters, but it wasn't at the bottom. They told me I had to have a wide excision, with substantial margins, and they would check what's called the sentinel node. They inject radioisotope around the lesion and then follow it for a couple of hours to see what lymph nodes it goes to. That was to be followed by a wide excision, and then the sentinel node would be biopsied to see whether there was any distant metastasis.

I had the surgery with a general surgeon and a plastic surgeon as well. They wanted to make sure I could still throw a baseball, so I had my hand up over my head when they put me to sleep. They biopsied the sentinel node and it had some cancer cells in it. There were no more cancer cells in the primary excision; they had left and gone to the lymph node.

You can read the total world's literature on melanoma in a couple of hours. There's a lot made of it; but as for the actual treatment, we don't have a real good answer. There are some people in Los Angeles who are using an immune vaccine type therapy, but I decided that if I was going to die, I wanted to die at home and not at UCLA. I'd never thought about death before. My body had never failed me in sixty-plus years, and I was kind of P.O.'d that it had now. I wasn't a happy camper.

We found a protocol that seemed to at least make sense. You use a drug called Tamoxifen, which is used in women's breast cancer. The concept was that you use the Tamoxifen to soften the melanoma cell, then you hit it with Cis-platinum, which is a potent chemotherapy agent, and then you use Interferon and Interleukin to pump up your immune system. You get three rounds of that, and it makes you pretty sick.

My amount of Tamoxifen was twenty tablets a day. A normal dose is one a day, so I would really get nauseated. We tried it in mashed potatoes, ice cream, crushing it, mashing it, and putting it in chocolate. Pretty soon it's like the Pavlovian response; you get sick just thinking about it. But it continued to work. It really made a lot of difference. I worked every day, except the three days I got the Cis-platinum. After three rounds of that, it either works or it doesn't. So far it has, and it's been three years.

If the tumor does come back, there are some newer things that are being used in Texas. Basically, the concept is that you take your tumor, work it out in a laboratory, teach it to become a killer cell, and look for its cousins. Then you inject it back in. Some people die of the treatment, so you want to be sure that you're treating the right disease.

I'm a cardiologist. Cardiology and oncology are a long ways apart, so I didn't know very much about melanomas. However, there isn't anything in medicine that's all that complicated, there's just a lot of it. You rely on the people who have been around you for a lot of years to at least give you sound advice and to make sure that you're not doing something stupid.

But, I think I am still unhappy because despite the fact that I have no family history of cancer, my body just failed me.

"One of five Americans will eventually develop melanoma or its less lethal cousins, basal cell and squamous cell carcinoma. From the year 2000 to 2001, the number of victims of melanoma jumped 9 percent. Yet, experts say, most people still shrug off warnings of the disease."

— *The Skin Cancer Institute,*
New York City

"I didn't think skin cancer was real cancer. But when you're handed a survival rate, it feels very real. I've reprogrammed my family for a whole new lifestyle. I make an extra effort to protect myself and them from the sun every day."

— *Shonda Schilling—melanoma,*
wife of Arizona Diamondback pitcher
Curt Schilling

Ellie Glaser—cancer of the lymph nodes
Forty-five years old—Del Mar, California
Working single parent

I had cancer in my lymph nodes under each arm. First I had radiation and then we progressed into chemotherapy. I had five different series of forty-five radiation treatments each, every day, Monday through Friday. Then I had two different sessions of chemotherapy. The first round was a series of twelve, and the second was a series of eight.

I was really tired, mostly from the process rather than from the procedure. It required having to go every day to the radiation center, waiting a little bit, and then having the treatment, which is actually very quick. But the process drains you. Nonetheless, I was very fortunate in that I was working full-time and never missed work because of my treatments. When I got into chemotherapy, I took Monday afternoons off for my sessions. Other than being extremely tired, I really didn't have many of the common side effects such as nausea. However, the radiation burned my skin. It becomes very, very sensitive, and some of the clothing I wore rubbed me the wrong way, which became very uncomfortable.

I strongly believe in mind over matter, and I was just absolutely convinced in my mind that I needed to keep life as normal as possible for my two children and me. I just believed that I'd go in, take care of business, and then come home.

I always told my doctor, "Don't tell me how many treatments I have remaining; just tell me when it's my last one." It seems inevitable that if you anticipate a stop time and you have to go a little bit longer, it becomes very difficult mentally because you think you're at the end, but you're not.

Then one day I came home and told my son, "Good news. This was my last treatment of chemo." He looked me in the eye and said, "Does that mean you're not going to be home on Monday afternoons?"

The basis for this question is that I had always worked extensive hours full-time, and it was rare if I was there when my kids got home from school.

During chemo, even though I may have been sleeping, I was home, which was a major happening. For him to say that put things in a lifetime perspective for me. From then on I changed. I decided I had to figure out a way to be home more when my kids come back from school.

That was a mental turning point for me. I was all excited that I was finishing something that was a bit of a hiccup in life's plan; but for my son, it was more important that he knew I was going to be there when he got home from school on Mondays. Even though I may have been sleeping, my body would still be there.

"To lift your spirits everyday do something for yourself. Take a walk on the beach, take a bubble bath, go to a movie, read a good book, or have a fabulous dinner. You deserve it."

— *Doris Ellsworth—non-Hodgkins lymphoma*

Maryann Rosenthal, Ph.D.

Fifty-four years old—La Jolla, California
Licensed clinical and consulting psychologist

My mother went into the hospital for what we thought was the flu. At eighty years of age, she still looked like a very healthy woman. She went into the hospital and they did all the tests. The doctor told my brother and me that she had pancreatic cancer and that it was so far along she was not going to live more than a few months. He then asked, "Who is going to tell her?" My brother said, "I'm not going to tell her." The doctor said, "Well, I'm not telling her." And I said, "Okay, I guess I'll tell her." So it was left up to me.

Their concern was if she knew she had cancer, she'd give into it and that would be the end. But I knew my mom, and I knew she was a feisty little Irish woman who could handle anything, if she knew what she had to deal with. I'm the same way; just tell me what it is and I'll make the adjustments.

So I sat on the side of her bed in the hospital, and she looked at me and said, "I don't have the flu, do I?" I said, "No, you don't have the flu. You're really sick, Mom." We just stared at each other, then I said, "I'm going to tell you straight up; you have pancreatic cancer, and the doctor says you don't have very long to live." She got really quiet, and I wondered whether she was going to cry or break down, but she was very calm. She looked at me and said, "Okay, all right." I said, "Are you afraid to die?" She thought about it for a minute but didn't answer quickly. Then she said, "No. I'm not afraid to die. I'm okay." And I knew she was going to be fine.

The chemo did not go well, she got really, really sick. During the second chemo, she was very sick again. Before she got off the table, she looked up at me and said, "I'd rather die. You know, I'm not afraid to die, and this is not quality living." I looked at the people who were giving her the chemo and said, "She's not going to have anymore chemo."

The doctor fought with me about that; he wanted her to go ahead with the chemo. But I said, "No." He said to me, "You're acting like you're God," which I thought was a very strange thing for a doctor to say. We got in an argument and I said, "In this instance, I am God; she's not having anymore chemo." I had no idea why he was so adamant about the fact that he wanted to give her chemo, but we stopped it and she went fairly quickly. She died with dignity, a very cool lady.

Arte Johnson—lymphoma, prostate cancer
Sixty-eight years old—Los Angeles, California
Actor—TV series Laugh In

The doctors found a tumor in my lungs. They didn't know what it was, but when they went in, it was lymphoma. So I had to fight that. I'm what you call a survivor.

Then I got nailed with another form of cancer that most men will encounter during the course of their lives—prostate cancer. The doctors also had to take that away. I have so many lines all over my body that you can use me as a road map.

During that entire period of time, I didn't ask too many questions. I didn't want to know; I just wanted to get it done with. My attitude was that this was just another step in my life.

I had my wife play jazz and Cuban music in the house. I didn't want any classical music because that was too down for me. I didn't want any books in the house that were serious or made me uncomfortable, just funny books with pictures.

I didn't do any cancer research because, I thought, what good would it do but confuse me. My wife once turned to the oncologist and asked, "Is he going to die from this?" The oncologist said, "No." Then I said, "That's all I wanted to hear. Don't give me a book to read about cancer, just stick a needle in me. Let's go, the faster the better."

I grew up being Tyrone, my "dirty old man" character on "Laugh In." Now I'm in my Tyrone years. I'm very excited about Tyrone. He shows that there is always hope, no matter how old you are.

I've ended up being a very successful guy. I look back on my life and am glad I had a chance to save for a rainy day. It's raining right now, and I'm having a ball.

"Cancer is truly an equal opportunity disease. It has no respect for any age group. I personally cannot comprehend my prostate cancer returning. If it rang the bell at my front door, I would tell it that all solicitors must go to the back door, and then I would get the hell out of Dodge."

— *Charlie Jones—prostate cancer,*
co-author

The Goodman Family
R.C., Dorothy, Cole, and Wyndal
Fort Smith, Arkansas

R.C. Goodman, M.D.—prostate cancer
Eighty-two years old
Retired anesthesiologist

I was sixty-eight years old (fourteen years ago) when I started my radiation. I went to St. Louis for a second opinion to see the man who developed the PSA test, Dr. William Catalona. He told me, "You have a large prostate gland. If I were sitting in your chair, I would have radiation." This is a doctor who operates on people all over the world and who developed the PSA, so I felt good about his recommendation, and I started my radiation. I continued to work. Some days I couldn't make it a whole day, but I continued to go every morning and try.

When they first told me I had cancer, it kind of changed my outlook on things. I don't know exactly how. I would say that emotionally it's more like a roller coaster. One hour I'd say, "Oh, what's the point?" and the next hour I'd say, "I'm going to lick this." You're up one hour, and you're down the next. There were times when I'd say, "I've got it, I've got to accept it, and I've got to cope with it." The word cope is what's important, the ability to cope with the situation. Some people cope with it a lot better than others and some people just go to pieces. I never went to pieces, but I certainly had second thoughts. I've always been very healthy, and I thought, This looks like it's fixing to catch up with me. Thank goodness it didn't, but that's the way I felt.

The first day I got home after I started forty-five days of radiation, I told Dorothy, "Well, 1/45th of that sucker is gone." The next day, I said, "Well, there's 2/45ths of it gone." Every day that they radiated me, I figured,

"Well, they just got a few more cells. There's certainly less in there than there was to begin with."

I get my PSA done on my birthday every year. I get concerned about it, but I don't go off the deep end and get real nervous like I used to. I figure at my age, 90 percent of men eighty-two years old have cancer cells in their prostate, but that's not the cause of their demise. They die with it, not because of it.

Dorothy Goodman—colon cancer
Seventy-nine years old
R.C.'s wife

The doctors never told me I had cancer. They said something was there and they had to see what it was. But any thinking person in this day and time would immediately think cancer. And I did. But, fortunately, I only had to wait from Thursday until Monday for surgery because they scheduled it immediately. So I didn't have a lot of time to worry about it.

It may sound strange to you, but I just prayed: "God, if it's cancer, let me be able to cope with it." I really did not get frantic or anything. I guess I very easily could have. But because R.C. was frantic for me, I didn't dare get upset too much. He gets awfully upset. In the end, he's very strong; but for me and our family, he gets very, very nervous.

I was so lucky because we caught it and it was contained. It was very large. They had to take out a third of my colon.

At the time I realized I probably had cancer, one of the best friends I've ever had in my life, Janie Saviers, was dying of cancer. I said to myself, "I hope that if I have cancer I can bear it as graciously as she has done." She was so lovely and so nice and loving to her family and friends. She was a real example to everyone.

Cole Goodman, M.D

Fifty-six years old
Plastic surgeon, son of R.C. and Dorothy,

My father is a prostate cancer survivor. My mother is almost a four-year colon cancer survivor. My brother Wyndal, the fourth boy, has metastatic renal cell cancer, which is a very bad form of cancer. He has been in the program at the National Institutes of Health (NIH). I was the bone marrow donor for him and I'll tell you, I'm really impressed with the NIH—and I'm a physician, as is my dad. We don't know if it's going to be successful, but Wyndal is hanging in there. He sure has been through a lot, but he's quite a trooper. Three weeks ago, he finished radiation therapy to his brain.

The way they're doing the harvest now for the stem cells is not bad at all. They hook you up to a machine, run your blood through it, and filter it. Each one of these cells in the blood has a different molecular weight, so they set the filter to whatever it is they're looking for. They take the lymphocytes, which are the immune system cells, first. That only takes three-and-a-half hours. You're in bed, and you can watch television or a movie. It's not that bad. The hard part for me was that the day they did my stem cells I had to stand up to "pee," and it's kind of hard to do that when your arms are straight. It's also difficult to do when there's a strange woman holding the plastic container. ·

The aphaeresis for the stem cells took almost six hours. Six days ahead of time, I started taking Granulocyte-Colony Stimulating Factor (G-CSF), and I gave it to myself sub-cutaneousely. It makes you feel bad—headaches, bone aches—especially in the hips. If you were doing it for another reason, it might be pretty bothersome, but it wasn't bothersome for me.

They wanted a minimum of three billion stem cells per harvest, and they had me scheduled for two harvests. They needed five billion to do the transplant. In one harvest I gave them 9.3 billion. My brother calls me the "Stem Cell Stud Muffin." I was pretty damn proud myself. By doing that, we didn't have to harvest the next day, so Wyndal and I had time to tour the Civil War battlefields. We both like history, especially Civil War and World War II history. That was one of the benefits of being able to be with him. He's a fine, fine man. He's the kindest human being I've ever known. He's very brave, but the odds aren't good.

Wyndal Goodman—renal cell carcinoma (kidney cancer)
Forty-eight years old
Environmental consultant, son of R.C. and Dorothy, and brother of Cole

I had renal cell carcinoma in my right kidney. I essentially found it in February 2001, when I could feel a mass right underneath my ribcage on my right side. After about a month of saying, "That doesn't really belong, what is that?" I asked my dad what he thought and he said, "Get your butt to the doctor."

My father, being the ultimate optimist that he is, thought that it might be my gall bladder, or something like that. I had the CT scan and they said, "You're going to have to have that kidney removed." So, I had my right kidney removed along with the tumor, which was fairly good size. However, the cancer had spread to my lymph nodes and to my adrenal gland, which they also removed during surgery.

At the time, I also had a couple of little spots on my lungs. They said they were too small to biopsy but the only way to know if it's a spread of the renal cell cancer was to keep an eye on it to see if it grows.

In November 2001, they said, "These things are getting bigger. You've got metastatic disease in your lungs." There's no such thing as a good cancer, but renal cell cancer is particularly tough. The renal system is your kidney and your bladder. The prognosis is particularly grim. Statistically, 75 percent of the people are dead within eighteen months of diagnosis. It's particularly resistant to traditional chemo and radiation therapies, and surgery may or may not be an option. It depends on where it is.

The oncologist who I went to had seen lots of failures using conventional therapies to treat renal cell cancer, and he told me, "You're too young. Conventional therapies are probably just going to put you through the wringer and not do anything for you." So he recommended I get into experimental research therapy at the National Institutes of Health (NIH) in Bethesda, Maryland, where they have an experimental stem cell transplant. Some of their renal cell patients are about five years out now. Their success rate is running about 60 percent as opposed to 15 percent for conventional therapies. So I said, "Sign me up!" In mid-February, I went to Bethesda, where I stayed until the end of June.

The stem cell transplant protocol calls for a donor who is a matched sibling. You don't get into the program unless you have a matching brother or sister as a donor. Cole was my donor. He was the best match.

The protocol is seven days of chemotherapy, essentially to knock my immune system down but not completely destroy it, which a lot of therapies will do. They call it a non-myelo-ablativ, which means the chemotherapy does not destroy bone marrow; all it does is knock down the white blood cell count. My white blood cell count essentially dropped to zero, which was their objective. At that point, they do the transplant. Cole had to be there for about two weeks to undergo various testing and screening to make sure he was physically up to the process.

I had the stem cell transplant in March 2002, in Bethesda. Their protocol said I had to agree to stay within a one-hour drive of the NIH, which is a huge facility. Everybody I came in contact with there was very professional, very compassionate, which impressed me. I was hospitalized as an in-patient for about four weeks. It was a week of chemotherapy followed by the stem cell transplant, and then the rest of the time was observation, because there was the possibility of complications. Just like any other transplant, there was the chance of rejection of foreign bodies in my body. I didn't have any complications from that, so they sent me home.

I got home on Sunday, June 30th, and on Wednesday morning, July 3rd, I woke up with a splitting headache. First, I tried to knock it down with Tylenol, but that didn't work. I went to my primary care physician. He gave me some morphine, but that didn't put a dent in the headache. They sent me to the emergency room where they gave me intravenous demerol, intravenous morphine, and oxycodone, and then said, "Nothing is helping this guy, we better do a CT scan on his head and see what's going on."

They did a CT scan and found I had metastatic disease in my brain. In other words, I've got kidney cancer in my brain. I don't have lung cancer; I have kidney cancer in my lungs. Two different beasties. Now I've got the brain tumors. They gave me mega doses of steroids to shrink the swelling, which took care of the headache. My local oncologist and the people at the NIH put their heads together and told me, "You need to have total brain radiation therapy."

For five weeks, five days a week, from Monday through Friday, I had radiation therapy, which is a total brain barbecue. As far as I'm concerned, it's the most diabolical medical treatment ever thought of by fat, bald guys in white lab coats. Total brain radiation was like they just dumped me in a black hole. I got to the point where I had no energy. I had a hard time getting up out of my chair just to walk across the room.

My mental faculties were affected in that I couldn't think or communicate easily. It affected my vision. Everything was wavy. I couldn't read or even watch TV. I also couldn't work, nor could I even get on the Internet. My wife had to read my e-mail, and I couldn't type to respond. I had no hand-eye coordination. It was the most God-awful thing I'd ever been through in my entire life. I also had a huge appetite through all of this, so I gained weight. If I wasn't sleeping, I was eating. Part of that was because I had the IV steroids in the hospital and then got on oral steroids (munchies).

I finished the radiation therapy on August 16th. I don't know if I'm talking coherently, but I'm at least able to carry on a conversation. Last Sunday, I was able to read the Sunday paper for the first time, and now reading the daily newspapers, which is a recent improvement.

Cancer is a waiting game. They'll do something, and you just have to wait and see. The hardest part for me to cope with is the waiting game. When I was at the NIH, I saw a lot of examples of success, and I was very optimistic and very positive. I believed then, and believe now, that the stem cell transplant and Cole's stem cells are going to beat this thing.

At the NIH, I would see six- and seven-year-old little kids running around with leukemia. They were an inspiration because they were fighters. Heads down, fists clenched, they were going to live. It also taught me the lesson to never ask, "Why me?" What I learned from those kids who haven't had a chance to do anything wrong and still got a hideous disease like leukemia was, don't give up! Fight this thing.

I'm trying to have as much fight in me as my parents do. You have to find that inner strength and draw on it. I've been married for fifteen years and I want at least fifteen more with my wife. I haven't gone fishing enough. There are so many things I still want to do. I got hammered during the radiation therapy and am just now starting to get my optimism back. In my case, for whatever reason, I don't think I could fight this very well without my family behind me.

"I learned never to say, 'The treatment is worse than the disease.'"

— *Wyndal Goodman*

"You gotta believe.'"

— *Tug McGraw—tumor covering both sides of the brain, quoting the rally slogan of the comeback New York Mets*

"When we first learned that I had colon cancer, my husband Ozzy became hysterical. The doctor had to come to the house and sedate him."

> — *Sharon Osbourne—colon cancer,*
> *Queen Bee of the MTV rock clan,*
> *The Osbournes, on her husband's*
> *reaction to her cancer*

"Don't ever attach this to my name. But I had my university friends bring me marijuana, and every afternoon I had marijuana tea. That helped me with the nausea."

> — *Cancer survivor,*
> *name withheld by request*

Chapter Three
Kids are Tough

This is the most difficult of all. Children should never have cancer. It should not happen to them, but it does. Cancer is not fair.

However, kids are much stronger than we realize. They have great courage. They fight to be individuals. Boy, are they tough! They don't want to be a number; they want to be seen as a person. One of the things we noticed about kids with cancer is how aware they are of other kids with cancer, and how they go about helping them. We can gain great insight by observing these youngsters.

In families where cancer has happened, we are constantly reminded of one thing, the strength and love of the mom and dad who immediately give up their own lives to battle for the life of their child.

"Briten was diagnosed with acute lymphocytic leukemia, cancer of the blood, on March 10, 1991. She was four years old. Now every March 10th we celebrate another anniversary of her being in remission. Which means, she's not cured; it just means that she's doing well."

— *Corinna Douglas,*
Briten Douglas's mom

John Mendelsohn, M.D.

Sixty-six years old—Houston, Texas
President of the University of Texas, M.D. Anderson Cancer Center

When a kid comes in with cancer, he or she comes into the environment of busy clinics and needles and treatments that sometimes hurt, and it can be terribly threatening and frightening. Our goal is to make the clinic environment friendly, empathetic, and supportive for the child and his or her parents. The parents are very, very important in this. If they have a positive attitude, that's half the battle.

At M.D. Anderson, we have two ongoing schools. The public school system pays for part of it, and we pay for part of it. A child gets classes that carry right along with whatever they were doing in school and, thus, the hospital becomes sort of a normal part of the routine instead of a place you go to instead of your normal place. A child can get used to all kinds of invasive threats if there's a warm and friendly hand and a sympathetic approach.

The people who take care of children often spend more time per patient and per procedure than they would with an adult, in order to play with the kids. The kids help each other tremendously. We have a little gym in our place and a big playroom, in addition to the school. The kids who have been through it will sit and talk with the new kids. They share and help support each other. Fortunately, the majority of childhood cancers are curable; unfortunately, not all are.

Stephen H. Friend, M.D., Ph.D.

Forty-nine years old—West Point, Pennsylvania
President of Rosetta Inpharmatics, Inc.; Vice President, Basic Research,
Merck Research Laboratories, Merck & Co., Inc.

I started out as a pediatric oncologist. I got to the point where I could not look into the eyes of the children because I knew when we started on some of those patients that they really weren't going to make it.

Of the drugs that we are using in cancer, nine out of ten of them are twenty to forty years old. It's a field that is not filled with the newest drugs such as the ones we have for lowering cholesterol, because the disease is so much more complex than anyone thought, and they have treated it as if it were very simple. That's what has driven me for the last fifteen years.

We have some advances that are now coming along. I want to be able to look into the eyes of some of those kids when we have something to offer them. I think I'm going to see that in the near future. I don't know what the timing is on all this because there is still work to be done. One drug we have is one that I'm looking at in terms of being close. It's not ready for open discussion yet but, hopefully, in the next six months to a year, we may be able to help some of those little kids.

Maryann Rosenthal, Ph.D.

Fifty-four years old—La Jolla, California
Licensed clinical and consulting psychologist

Kids are strong. They are really tough. A lot of the time, the kids I've dealt with who have had cancer have taken a different approach to it than the adults. I don't think their mortality becomes an issue. They're just there. Talk about being in the present, they're going to take the next step. That's their attitude. They're fearless. Adults who have cancer get in a trapped mode. Their fear traps them and keeps them trapped.

Part of the difference is the fact that the older you become, the more you feel you have to lose, because you've had more experiences. A seven- or eight-year-old kid is not losing sons, grandsons, and granddaughters. Mentally, they haven't gotten to that. Their world is much smaller.

I was involved in treating a group of kids who were really far along in their cancer. After they went through some treatment and some sessions, we threw a dance for them. It was a costume party, or so I thought. I seemed to be the only one who dressed up in a costume. I guess I didn't get the memo. I came all decked out like a disco queen. I'll never forget the costume; it was awesome. I still have pictures of it.

It was all really fun, and this one little boy, who was just a pistol, came up and looked at me and I said, "Come on, let's dance." He took another look and said, "You're just too weird, I'm not dancing with you." He turned around and walked away and I thought, Here's this little kid, baldheaded and just a mess, and he's telling me I'm weird. But it was great, because as he walked away, he had the biggest grin on his face.

Briten Douglas—acute lymphocytic leukemia
Fifteen years old—Escondido, California
Sophomore in high school

I was four years old when I got acute lymphocytic leukemia, cancer of the blood. I remember almost everything because it made such an impact on my life that it's really hard to forget. I'll start from the very beginning.

I was born with bladder extrophy. What that means is I was born without a bladder; it was outside of my body, and I had no pelvic bone. The doctors had to reconstruct me from birth. So I was basically living at the hospital all the time. The doctors said, "If she lives, she won't be able to walk." But through everything, I was finally able to walk. I was always at the doctor's office getting different things done. The doctors and nurses were like my second parents.

Then one night when I was four, I went to bed and I woke up with this really, really sharp pain in my tummy. It felt like a knife that just kept stabbing me in the gut. I ran into my parent's room in tears saying, "Please take me to the doctor. I need to get this knife out of my tummy." They took me to the emergency room where they took a blood sample. Then after a little bit, they transferred us over to the hospital. The doctor came in and diagnosed me, but he didn't tell me the results. He took my parents outside and told them. Then they came back inside. It didn't really hit me at first. My parents just said, "Okay, we're going to have to keep coming back to the hospital."

From that point on, everything changed. I had to get treated right then and there. They put a Hickman, a catheter that went straight to my heart, in my chest. And day after day, week after week, I'd have to return for chemotherapy. I lost my hair. But that was really cool. It was my favorite thing. I liked the look. They bought me a tricycle that I could put my little IV on, and I loved riding it around the playroom at the hospital.

What else I remember are my friends. I was supposed to start kindergarten, but I had to wait a year because I wasn't allowed to be around anybody who had chickenpox or any other kind of sickness because even catching a cold could be life threatening to me.

Another cool thing was when the child life specialists would bring in visiting dogs, because I wasn't allowed to have any pets during my three-year treatment. However, as soon as my treatment was over, my parents stopped off at an animal place where they got me a cat. I named her Remi for remission, and I've been in remission for eleven years now. Unfortunately, Remi ran away about a year ago.

I can never forget having to go in and sit on the edge of a bed and wait and wait until finally the nurse would come in and give me a leg shot or take me into the back room for a spinal tap. Those are painful things you just can't forget. Throwing up day and night, just throwing up everything, was seriously the norm for me. Taking pills. Oh, my gosh, day and night, oral pills around the clock. It was just horrible. They would give me about ten every day. It was just crazy. And I'd have to swallow them.

I remember learning to swallow pills when I was four years old. They taught me how by putting M&Ms in vanilla ice cream. I'd take a bite of vanilla ice cream and then have to swallow the M&Ms. I'd say, "Oh, it's an M&M, yummy!" I would chew the M&Ms so when they finally put the real pill in the vanilla ice cream, I chewed that too. It was the type of medicine that was unbelievably gross. Like something you would die over because it was so nasty. To this day, I cannot eat vanilla ice cream because I remember taking that one bite into a big, fat, white pill that just totally destroyed vanilla ice cream forever. But that's how I learned to swallow pills.

One of my nurses was really nice. She felt really bad when she had to give me my first leg shot because it was so scary and it hurt really bad. In fact, she felt so bad for having to do that to me that she let me give her a shot of saline in her arm. I actually got to do that. I played nurse. She was really neat. All the nurses and doctors were very supportive. And they still are whenever I go in for my checkups. They always say hi to me and ask me how I'm doing. It's just like my second family and my second home.

When I had to stay in the hospital for a week or two, they would put me in a room with another kid. You know, you have one TV and stuff like that and there are two families in this itty-bitty room. I'd always make friends with those kids who were brought in with cancer. We'd become friends and then one morning I'd wake up and wonder, "Where did my friend go?" My friend got taken away because she or he had passed away in the night. When I would make friends, it wouldn't be for very long because normally, they wouldn't make it. Reality would hit me and I'd think, Am I going to die? I could die, too. Why aren't I dying? Everybody else is. And then I'd attend their funerals. I attended so many funerals at a very young age, that I felt like death was just waiting right there at my doorstep.

I really didn't have a lot of outside friends because I wasn't allowed to go to school or to be very social. That was kind of hard. People were really scared. They would distance themselves from my family, not wanting to be near me because I had cancer. They didn't want to be affiliated with that at all. That was disappointing.

Right now I have a lot of friends all over the place. I like to be very outgoing and meet as many people as I can. It's something that I didn't really have before. I don't regret anything. I don't have any regrets at all. I wouldn't take back having cancer because it has opened so many new doors for me. I'm allowed to go to cancer camp, and they hold special functions to honor cancer patients and things like that. I'm able to speak to many different charities to help raise money to find a cure for cancer someday. So, actually, what happened to me is a very positive thing in my life.

I definitely want to go to college. Actually, I'm thinking about becoming an anesthesiologist or a lawyer. Not like a criminal lawyer or anything like that. I don't want a mean job at all. I have to be very nice. Being an anesthesiologist, I could help people understand the point of view of the kids. Many doctors have no clue about what's going on. They just do their best with their book knowledge, procedure after procedure.

I'd be very social with the kids and understand what they're going through because I went through that, too. But my most sky-high goal out of everything is I want to be somebody famous, like a famous actress, a movie star. I want to win an Oscar. That would really be cool. It's the highest goal of my life. I'm already working on my acceptance speech.

Guy Miller—leukemia

Thirty-two years old—Poway, California
Second grade teacher, at age sixteen, diagnosed with acute leukemia. Underwent
chemotherapy from April 7, 1986 to July 21, 1988 (two years, three months).

During that two-plus years I was going through chemotherapy, there were times when I would wonder if it was really worth it. As I look back now, I think it was the fear of the unknown that kept me going.

What would happen if I stopped? What was it like to die? What was it like for my friends who had leukemia when they passed away? Were they in pain?

You come to grips that it's okay to die, but the fear of not knowing what it's going to be like; not where you're going to go, but how you're going to get there, keeps you alive. It can be a bit schizophrenic. There are two people inside you battling it out. You have to be sure that the positive you outweighs the negative you.

There was a point in time during my treatment, about halfway through, when I was home alone, sitting in our big Lazy Boy recliner. My friend Hugo had just died, and my friend Norma had died a few weeks before that. I was due for more chemo. It was one of those sessions that would make me throw up until I fell asleep that night, so that meant I'd be throwing up for six hours straight. My mom came home from work, and I spun around and looked at her and said, "I'm done. I'm ready to die. I can't take the chemo anymore."

I had the faith that I knew I'd be going to heaven. I knew I'd be better off there. I wouldn't be in anymore pain, and I wouldn't be throwing up all the time. The worst part of chemo is not only looking different, but also the nausea, not being able to do some of the things you want to do, and the uncertainty of your fate.

When I told my mom I was ready to go, she put down her stuff. She was a rock. She sat down and said, "You can't do that. You can't give up. This is your battle. We're here for you, but this is your battle. You can't give up."

She told me that if I gave up it would be almost like a form of suicide, which is a selfish thing because there are so many people who love you and care for you and want to do whatever they can for you. To give up would be a slap in their face since they're doing everything they can for you. Then we prayed together.

_____

"I was a teenager who happened to be a leukemia patient, not a leukemia patient who happened to be a teenager."

— *Motto adopted by Guy Miller's family*

Charles B. "C.B." Wolford—Ewing's sarcoma (a rare form of cancer that starts in the bone tissue and spreads throughout the skeletal system)
Thirteen years old—Phelps, Kentucky
Seventh grade student

Sometimes I cry myself to sleep. I wonder, why me? Why did it have to happen to me? But I guess I am just as good a choice as anybody. If it hadn't happened to me, it would have happened to somebody else. You just have to keep your faith. That's what kept me hanging on. Maybe I will get better and everything will go back to normal.

I wanted to try a new experimental chemotherapy. Even if it didn't help me, they might find out something new by experimenting on me. It might save another child. Then my life would mean something to some other family.

Faye Wolford
Mother of C.B., who died fourteen months after being diagnosed with Ewing's sarcoma. He was fourteen years old.

All of C.B.'s friends were so kind to him. As soon as they found out he had cancer, all the boys shaved off their hair so he wouldn't feel bad about being bald due to his chemo. I thank the Lord every day that there are still people in this world who care about other people's feelings.

C.B. said he was going to beat cancer and, in a way, he did. The cancer died with him. He won his battle the only way he could. At least I know I now have an angel in heaven who is looking out for me.

Ballard Wolford
C.B.'s dad

When C.B. woke up on the last morning of his life, I put a tape in the VCR and we watched it together. That day feels like a dream to me. I don't remember ever leaving his side. When he died that night, I couldn't make myself move away from his bed. I just kept saying, "He's not dead. He can't be. It's not supposed to happen this way." But it did.

I didn't know why I lost my child and I probably won't ever know. I do know that a piece of me died that day. The only thing that keeps me going is my other son Eddie. I know he needs me more now than he ever did. All I cared about were my two sons.

Eddie Dean Wolford
C.B.'s brother

The day I found out my brother had cancer was the worst day of my life. I was so scared for C.B. and for myself. I was afraid that if he had cancer, I would have it too. All I knew about cancer was that it would kill you in the end, and that scared me to death.

I hope that everyone who has a brother is as lucky as I was, because my brother was an angel here on earth, just as I know he is now up in heaven. I love you C.B., and I always will until the last breath leaves my lungs.

(Courtesy of author, excerpts from *My Story About Cancer*)

Alden Seabolt—Burkitt's lymphoma

Fifteen years old—Atherton, California
Freshman in high school

I was diagnosed with Burkitt's lymphoma, and then I had a CNS (central nervous system) relapse. There are two different types of Burkitt's. The first is an African type that usually comes in the form of a tumor in the jaw. The second is a non-African type, which I had, that usually is around the intestinal area. I was fourteen at the time.

I was diagnosed at stage two, so I had three rounds of chemo. I puked a bit. I generally did not feel good, and my hair fell out. Then they discovered more cancer in my spine. There were cancer cells in my spinal fluid. So I had nine doses of Methotrexate, a chemotherapy agent, injected into my spine. It hurt quite a bit. Following that, I had a bone marrow transplant. My brother Garrett was the donor. Now I'm still in isolation. I get a check-up every week. I can't go into buildings, but the good news is I have no more chemo.

I have a lot of close friends. They visited me almost every day in the hospital, which helped brighten me. I put my trust in God. I believed He would do the right thing and that He would heal me. With a positive attitude, everything went pretty smoothly. My friends can now come over, as long as they're completely healthy and they wash their hands.

I go to the Children's Hospital at Stanford University—the Lucile Packard Hospital. There is a school there, and I get to work outside with the teachers. Basically, whoever is an inpatient at the hospital, or whoever is in the hospital for an extended period of time and can't otherwise get schooling, is allowed to attend. They have private tutors who follow the curriculum from the school you normally attend. I still go to the hospital for school.

I want to complete high school, and I don't know where I want to go to college, but I would either like to be a business major or a veterinarian major. I'm really interested in animals. I try to think positively; otherwise, I get kind of depressed, which doesn't make anything better.

Steve Seabolt
Alden's father

Somehow Mike Ovitz, in Los Angeles, heard about Alden and that we were trying to get into the UCLA Medical Center. He's heavily involved in their fundraising. We don't know Mike Ovitz, but we do know he went out of his way to help a fifteen-year-old cancer patient. He was quite sincere in helping us in anyway he could. We ended up not going to UCLA, but his personal help is greatly appreciated.

Kyle Speer—leukemia (twice)
Five years old—San Marcos, California

I got leukemia not that long ago. I got well and then I got it again. Then I got rid of it again. I'm in remission, but they're still treating me. I don't have radiation. I just have chemotherapy.

I lost all of my hair. That was kind of fun because now I don't have to wash my hair all the time. When I found out I had leukemia the second time, I was in the hospital on my birthday. It is really neat to be in the hospital on your birthday because you get a lot more presents.

———————

"Kyle has a great attitude. For him, this has just been a part of his life. He's really honest and upbeat, and I think he enjoys the attention he gets. He finds a way to look at the good in things. He doesn't dwell, he just keeps moving on. He's pretty perky."

— *Carol Speer,*
Kyle's mother

Jennifer Thornton
Thirty-five years old—Boca Raton, Florida
Executive Director, The A-T Children's Project for Ataxia-Telangiectasia

The A-T Children's Project for Ataxia-Telangiectasia was founded by Brad and Vicki Margus in 1993, when they discovered that two of their boys were diagnosed with this disease. Because it's an extraordinarily rare disease, they didn't get the right diagnosis for a long time. It's a terrible disease because it's progressive. They had thought that one of their sons had mild cerebral palsy, but when they found out it was neuro-degenerative, killing the brain cells and predisposing them to cancer, and that it was often fatal by the late teens, they were devastated.

Children are born with A-T. It's genetic; both parents have to be carriers. Oftentimes, it's first noticed in kids when they are about two years old, because parents think their child appears a little bit too wobbly. Sometimes, they've been sick a lot with immune system problems and frequent colds and infections. They're often misdiagnosed with mild cerebral palsy. Many times, things can be relatively stable until the age of four, five, or six, when walking becomes more difficult and the child shows more signs of ataxia.

Because it's such a rare disease, very little research was being done on it, so the Marguses felt it was time to do specific research for it. They set up a foundation in 1993, which is this organization; started talking with other families coping with this disease and with children diagnosed with it; and started giving money to the foundation thinking that they were going to make advances happen.

Brad Margus is just an incredible man. He learned absolutely everything he could about the disease, and about what could be done. He banged on doors and wrote letters, faxed and called people, and wouldn't take no for an answer. He established a scientific advisory board to review grants. He raised money so researchers could start working on this disease. In ten years, we have been able to fund millions of dollars of research directly for A-T, and we have captured the attention of researchers all over the world.

It is a very interesting gene and we are finding how it relates to cancer and cancer risk in the general population, and how this gene and protein interact with cancer.

We're still looking for a cure for A-T. We raise about two million dollars a year. We spend it on research and on awareness activities and family support. We answer their questions, send them information, and help them get to the A-T Clinical Center at Johns Hopkins, which we established in 1995.

The research is very exciting, although we don't actually have any treatments yet. In the not so distant future, we're hoping to have some clinical trials, to try various compounds and anti-oxidants that might be able to stop the progression of the disease. We're also funding research in areas of gene therapy, neurostemso transplantation, and molecular biology. We're making progress, but I can't say we have anything yet that actually works to stop it. However, there is very, very promising progress on a lot of different fronts.

Ernie and Maria Schimmer

Laguna Hills, California

Parents of Ernest Schimmer (thirteen years old) who has Ataxia-Telangiectasia

The disease our son Ernest has is called Ataxia-Telangiectasia. We both have the defective gene. There are 500 kids in the United States who have it. A lot of them don't live past twenty years of age. There are thirty-five to forty in wheelchairs, and a couple of them are moving around okay. This defective gene affects your balance and makes you susceptible to leukemia.

We knew something was wrong with Ernest when he was about three years old and he was starting to wobble. He was playing soccer and he'd swing his foot and the ball had already gone by.

We took him to a physical therapist, who told us, "Don't worry about it. He'll be fine in a few months." He was diagnosed with dyskinesia, an unknown cause for balance problems. A couple of years later we were starting a new therapy through California Children's Services and they asked us if we wanted to see a neurologist. We did and she said, "There is more here than what you think." They did a blood test, and his immune system was not normal. They did an alpha-fetoprotein test, which is a liver enzyme. It was extremely high and that's how they diagnosed him with Ataxia-Telangiectasia. That's his genetic condition.

It was devastating because at the time, all the literature we had said that these kids do not make it past puberty. They die young and have all sorts of cancer. It was the most horrible week of our lives.

Then in 1997, a week after school had started, Ernest came home and said, "I don't want to go to school anymore." That surprised us, because Ernest always liked school. He said, "Those stairs are just too big for me to go down to the playground."

A few months later, we were combing his hair and saw two big lumps on the side of his throat. It didn't look good, so we took him to the pediatrician right away, and they immediately did all sorts of tests, including blood tests. The doctor called and said, "I'm not supposed to tell you this now, but it's leukemia. I've already called the hospital. Take him there as soon as possible because his white blood count is very high."

He was eight years old when he started chemotherapy. He did very well during treatment because we were giving him a lot of nutrition. He never had that dark murky look in his face; he never lost his hair. They just couldn't believe it. He was doing fine until 1999. We were so happy because his counts were improving and he was playing in the backyard on the monkey bars and said, "Look, I can do this again."

We'll never forget the date, it was August 6th. We went to the hospital for a check up and a spinal tap. We were getting ready to leave and the nurse came in and said, "The doctor wants to talk with you." She said, "He relapsed. It's in his central nervous system." He had never had leukemia in the central nervous system; it was all in his bone marrow. That was another blow. We couldn't find a treatment for Ernest. He could not have radiation because of his Ataxia-Telangiectasia. The doctors searched all over and found a treatment that required putting a shunt into his head and delivering the chemo directly with the shunt.

We did that, and then he became very tired and started throwing up. He was diagnosed in August, and they put the shunt in at the end of September. Then in late October, he was still throwing up and we just couldn't figure out why. On Halloween, we were sleeping with him and he kind of called us. He made a sound because he couldn't talk, and we saw him staring at us and knew something was wrong. We couldn't set him upright, he was stiff.

We rushed him to the emergency room. They were going to transfer him to the ICU, and we overheard the nurse telling the doctor, "They want to know why you want to transfer him to ICU." And the doctor replied, "This child is dying." He had massive brain damage because of the chemo, and no one usually recovers from this. The neuro surgeon came in and said, "There is nothing we can do. He's going to die. You can stay here or go home." We decided that if we went home we'd be closer to the family. We took him home with three antibiotics and all the medicines. It was round the clock nursing.

In November, Ernest was still here and we told the doctors, "He's coming back. He's saying something. He's . . . " But they didn't believe us. Then one day he opened his eyes a little bit when we were at the hospital. He started talking, but the doctors still didn't believe us. After the coma, we just knew he was going to stay alive. We never gave up on him. We just talked and talked to him. We'd tell him we'd take him to Disneyland and to Legoland when he got better. We started to do a lot of praying and we had Hawaiian healers and Indian healers. He was a whole month in the hospital, and they still thought he wasn't going to make it. He had constant fevers for three months.

They couldn't find anything wrong with him, so we asked a healer to come to the hospital. He checked his pulse and gave him a homeopathic remedy. He said that within forty-eight hours Ernest would have no more fever. Within forty-eight hours, the fever was gone. We left the hospital and haven't been back since. It's been a long road but he's getting better. We've always done alternative therapies and now we've started a new therapy in Encinitas, a sound therapy that has been working great.

Ernest is here for a purpose. We don't know the purpose yet, but he's recovering. He's mentally here. For the longest time he didn't talk, then one morning last year he started talking in full sentences. He goes to school. He's happy, everybody loves him. He's the star of the school.

We get the *Los Angeles Times*, and every day it has a children's section with jokes in it. Ernest cuts out a joke and takes it to school. The kids at his school, first and second graders, go to the library and say, "Where's Ernest? We want to hear his joke." He's getting so many awards for making a difference at school because of his patience and his will to learn.

Ernest is like a magnet, and people just look at him. We don't know why; of course, he is our child and we love him, but he has an extra something. He's very kind and cares about people. Everyone falls in love with him. He's a very handsome boy. That's how he ended up on TV with the program on the Learning Channel. They just looked at him, and said, "Can we follow him around?" It's been an odyssey, and he's still recuperating. It's not finished yet. He's a miracle child.

"A cigarette in the hands of a Hollywood star on screen is a gun aimed at a twelve- or fourteen-year-old. My hands are bloody and so are Hollywood's. Smoking should be as illegal as heroin."

> — *Joe Eszterhas—throat cancer, Hollywood screenwriter apologizing for putting so much smoking in his movie scripts such as* Basic Instinct, *where Sharon Stone and Michael Douglas were smoking in almost every scene*

Jim Canton

Thirty-six years old—Ashford, Connecticut
Executive director, Hole In The Wall Gang Camp

At Hole In The Wall Gang Camp, we completed our fifteenth summer in 2002, and we've had about 12,000 kid campers. We'll have over 1,000 in the summer of 2003. We have either six-day or eight-day sessions. We see children with cancer and other blood disorders, hemophillia, sickle cell anemia, HIV, and AIDS.

About 30 percent of our children have cancer, 25 percent have sickle cell, and 25 percent have HIV; the rest have rare blood disorders. We have a medical facility in camp and a team of nurses and doctors, so the children can get their chemotherapy here. They get whatever they need in order to keep them strong and enable them to enjoy the activities.

We modify all our programs so that we can give an all-inclusive experience to every child and give them an idea of what a healthy child would experience at a sleep-away camp. We try to return a sense of normalcy to their lives and remind them they're just kids. We let them do things that children should be able to do.

We also run programs throughout the year. We have twenty weekends out of the fall and spring where we try to reunite the children or serve their whole families or just have weekend retreats for the parents at the camp. In the winter when we can't run the camp, we go to the hospitals and clinics, visit our campers, and hold reunions.

When I first came to the camp, I was in the cabins, and it was absolutely humbling to see how courageous and resilient the kids are, and how much they just want to be kids. Give them a safe space to be rowdy, and they delight in it. The sharing they have with one another is phenomenal. If you say they are just children who want to be kids, that's true, but to only see that and to not see the bonds they share and the common language and sensitivity they have for one another's struggles, is doing them a disservice.

They are children who have been really sensitized. I think that's where their wisdom and courage come from. It is special how they can share that with one another. In my role now as executive director, I do whatever I can to get back into the cabins. I'll still volunteer two sessions in the cabins.

I can remember the very first summer. We had a child who had to go to the infirmary and missed out on a day of activities. I had a cabin of ten-year-old boys and among themselves, they decided to rotate out of activities throughout the day and go keep him company. Totally on their own, they decided to take some time out to visit with him. They would just say, "Can you take me to the infirmary? I want to go see Jimmy."

They're ready to do mischief as well. We've got campers who people have been so careful with that this is the first time they can finally be kids. I think we see these children sometimes better than their families do. They are free. We create a safe environment for them and have clear boundaries, but boy, can they play.

That's the whole point of the camp. It's not about doing therapeutic reflections or processing sessions, it's about learning how to canoe, fish, and ride a horse, in addition to discovering things about yourself that you never thought you could do. It's about getting in touch with what other children get in touch with all the time. In the past, these kids have been restricted from that, and with the camp experience, the result is just elation. Pride and self-esteem blossom in front of you.

When I tell people about camp, they say, "Oh, that must be such a sad place," but oh my gosh, it's just the opposite. It's so joyful to be a part of that healing process and to see it happen. It's pretty hard to explain. I wish I could bring people to it more often, but we want to let the kids have their time. We don't want them negatively affected by having folks circulating when all the magic is going on. Even the parents are not allowed. Camp allows time for kids to taste independence, and for their families to have some rest.

Some of these children have never been separated from their parents, so the issue of homesickness can be acute. We try everything we can to help. We try to be creative and resourceful and look for something they can hold onto. I've had a dog at camp for a couple of years, a yellow lab named Ripley, and he has more than earned his keep by easing homesickness. The families also experience separation anxiety, and we've spent hours with parents who are crying on the phone because they are so nervous and it's so painful to be separated from their child.

Camp gives kids a chance to stand out, and at the end of our sessions, we have an awards ceremony. We'll have 120 children per session for nine sessions over the course of the summer, and every single child will be called up individually to receive an award on stage for excelling in a certain program area. We do it quickly, so that the evening doesn't last four hours, but every child gets his or her own applause.

We have Stage Night the evening before the awards ceremony. When they come on stage, it's the greatest metaphor for the transformation that happens at camp. After you've seen them just eight days previously behaving so cautiously and guarded and then watch them come on stage before their peers and in front of a theater filled with 200–250 people and slowly start to sing a song or do a skit, it's amazing.

You see them start to relax as they hear the laughter and support of their friends and the clapping from the audience to the rhythm of the song. You see them just starting to take it in, and as they do, they are blossoming. So by the end of the act, when we force them to take a bow, they are drinking in all this applause. You can count on a standing ovation for the acts. We just want the kids to enjoy the moment and leave fuller.

The entire camp is built on builder statements. We say that camp is a place where everyone should feel safe, respected, and loved. There are three camp rules: (1) No physical violence; (2) No unsupervised activities; (3) No killer statements. Killer statements are things we say to someone to tear them down. Instead, we believe in builder statements, words to boost someone up. We tell the staff to take every opportunity that we can to feed that self-esteem in the sense of self-respect of each child by recognizing small victories. It's all about celebrating small victories.

The camp was Paul Newman's dream. He's the founder. He started this baby, and now he's responsible for the growth throughout the country and overseas. It's his vision. After he started his food company, Newman's Own, he never expected such success, so he decided to give away all of the company's profits to established charities.

He began to receive pleas from families saying, "My child is very sick. Would you please send us to Florida to Disney World?" Paul said, "Why don't we create a space where all these children can escape their sickness and be reminded of a childhood without illness?" So he created Hole In The Wall Gang Camp, with the name coming from his movie, *Butch Cassidy and the Sundance Kid*.

We tell children that like Butch and Sundance, who were able to find a safe space to enjoy their friendship, Hole In The Wall Gang Camp is a private space where they can feel safe, respected, and loved. As they come through the camp gates, all the things that are chasing them on the outside, stay outside.

We don't charge anything for the sessions, weekends, or services we provide. Everything is free of charge for the children and their families. We raise the money throughout the year. Our development office will raise five million dollars, plus additional amounts for any capital projects.

Many people think Paul Newman and Newman's Own underwrite the camp, and because they are good friends, they would be here if we needed them. However, after the first year when Newman's Own and Paul provided the seed money for the camp, they stepped away. They said, "Don't rely on us. Get your own development team together and raise your own funds." So that's what we've been doing, and there are now nine Hole In The Wall Gang Camps around the world.

Paul Newman

Seventy-eight years old
Founder, talked about Hole In The Wall Gang Camp with Pam Janis of
InTouch Cancer *magazine . . .*

As I got into my sixties, I began to really think about luck—how it works, who has it, who doesn't. As one book put it, children with cancer don't have a lifetime to correct bad luck or wait for it to change. We had the idea for the camp, but no credentials to build or run it. I made several false starts, looked at the wrong places. The most important ingredient we found was Doc Howard Pearson of Yale, a pediatric oncologist. Without the credentials he brought to this, we couldn't have gotten anywhere.

At first, very few people would trust us with their kids. The first session we had was only half full. I was standing out there in the driveway, waiting for people to show up, but they were not about to release their children to an untested, untried place. It was like being ready to throw a party and then hardly anyone coming. It wasn't until the very end of the summer that the word spread that this camp was an okay place, and that it was a safe place. That's when we knew we were on our way.

When I visited some other camps for children who were ill, I wasn't able to figure out from the looks of things what difference there was between the camp and the hospital. So I tried to create something that would have a sense of romance for kids and a sense of adventure.

We have a counselor for every two campers; increasingly, every year we've been able to take children who would be less likely for any kind of camp experience. We can do that because our medical staff has grown, which increases our ability to deal with chemotherapy and other treatments. There are no mandatory activities. Children can generally pick what they want to do, anything from handicrafts to theater to fishing.

It's my memory that one summer, they caught 11,000 fish up there. They can't keep them; they have to release them. The poor lips of the fish were so sore; they'd probably been caught fourteen or fifteen times. They're the only ones who are glad when the summer is over.

We have a gymnasium. We have rope climbs. We have horses. And let me tell you, we have a loud and noisy bunch of kids up there. It's loud and noisy and they raise hell and that's terrific. We have children who tell us that anticipating the week in the summer that they will be at camp is what keeps them going all year.

The kids think I'm the guy on the lemonade container. One summer when I was sitting with some of them in the mess hall, a little guy asked me if it was true I was a movie star. "I've made a few pictures," I said. He looked at me and said, "Man, them movies sure make you look young."

Julia Roberts volunteered up there—what a dynamite lady she is. A lot of people volunteer at the camp, too, but I tell this story because some little kid called her mother and said, "Mommy, Mommy, guess who I've got in my cabin? Tinker Bell!"

(Paul Newman's interview is reprinted with permission from The Oncology Group (formerly PRR, Inc.). Copyright 2001, *InTouch* 3 (1) : 26-28, 2001.)

"When I'm in the dumps, I come up here to Hole In The Wall Gang Camp, and it reaffirms everything I think is really good and generous about this country."

> — *Paul Newman,*
> *actor, founder, and CEO of Newman's Own, which gives all its after-tax profit to charity—more than $125 million and counting*

Andrea Jaeger

Thirty-seven years old—Aspen, Colorado
Former tennis great and co-founder of Silver Lining Ranch and
Kids Stuff Foundation

Kids don't come to Silver Lining Ranch to get cured of cancer. They come here to have life. We show them something inside themselves that perhaps they never thought was there, and that is: "I can do this. I can go to the top of Aspen Mountain. I can ride a horse on my own. I can raft down a river." When you're lying in a hospital bed, these things become very important.

Actually, these kids are giving us a gift. They're giving us the appreciation of life. They don't want to be a statistic; they don't want to be a number. They have names, they have faces, and they have courage beyond what you could ever imagine.

I want to tell you about Rhea. Rhea was one of the teenagers in the first group we ever had at Silver Lining Ranch. She was from Chicago, and she made a big impression on the entire staff. There's a huge difference between young children and teenagers. Teenagers understand a lot more about boyfriends and girlfriends and marriage and careers and having kids. So, when they're diagnosed with cancer, they think a lot more is being taken away from them than just their family.

Rhea came to Aspen wearing a wig. If you didn't work with kids with cancer you probably wouldn't have noticed it. She would tell us how frustrating it was that a lot of people didn't understand what she was experiencing. At her job, they didn't even believe she was going through chemotherapy, and they didn't want to give her days off because she looked so normal. Her spirit was incredible. She was going through all this, fighting for her life, and yet she was enjoying every moment. She understood what it was like not to know if you have tomorrow, so she was embracing today.

We were also dealing with younger children, and the differences were very obvious because Rhea was going through the same thing yet she was helping the younger kids in the session. When it was time for Rhea to leave, she began explaining to us how she pushed grocery carts in and out of a grocery store in Chicago during the midnight shift to earn money for gas to put in her mom's car to go take chemo. That's when we decided we were going to hire Rhea. We just didn't know what her job would be.

We called her as soon as she got home and said, "Look, we're going to be doing some different things. We can do a children's hospital newsletter that you can write and print and send out to hospitals for free. You can help us with different projects because you understand cancer; you're living with it so why not use that in terms of helping other families?" Rhea was just screaming; she was so excited she couldn't believe it. So that's what we did in the four years we had Rhea.

She taped a video to show what happens with cancer over the course of time. She took us into the hospital, introduced her nurses, and talked with people in the hallways. She then videotaped herself while she was taking her chemo. Each hour, as the chemo was being administered, you could see the changes. She started getting really sick. The color in her face would change. She'd start throwing up. She'd be crying. She threw off her wig. She was throwing up so much you could see the strain on her body. Eventually, she just had to turn off the camera.

Every child touches you in a certain way but because Rhea was in our first group, she taught us so much. She would tell us how a lot of people don't even understand what it's like not to have hair, especially having no eyebrows. That looks different. It looks freakish. She would explain things that happened to her during chemotherapy so that someone who never had dealt with the disease in that capacity would understand what a person has to live through. Here was someone who knew what she was dealing with and living with (we never say dying with), and helping us understand in greater detail so we could do more to help the other kids.

After four years of being part of Rhea's life, and Rhea being a part of the Foundation family, the cancer went into her bones. She'd gone through a remission and then she relapsed; there was nothing else the doctors could do. It's a silent policy that we don't go to funerals because if we did, we'd be going to a lot of them. (You can't just all of a sudden have the whole staff pack up and leave for a funeral service.)

Rhea called and tried to make me promise I would come to her funeral. She had gotten the diagnosis this time, and it was only a matter of months. She didn't want to know the exact time, but her mom told me it wasn't months, it was a matter of days. So I flew to Chicago. Rhea lived in a trailer home that had holes in the ceiling, yet she had never, ever complained. To see that and to see the way she dealt with death as honorably as the way she dealt with life, was amazing. It was something you can't even imagine, and she was still so young, just going on twenty-one.

I stayed with her a couple of nights in her trailer. I slept on the couch. The cancer was eating away at her in such drastic ways. I'd sit with her in the morning and talk with her, and do the same in the afternoon. She'd have broken blood vessels in her eyes or in her legs. She'd be struggling to breathe when she talked. She couldn't walk well. She didn't eat. I'd come in her room and she'd say, "Hey, do you want something from my closet? We're about the same size, you can have some of my clothes." I'd just sit there and think, How is she doing this? In a remarkable way, she was trying to give strength to all of us who cared for her.

One time she looked at me. We were just sitting and talking and she said, "Everyone will forget me." This was in one of her darker moments. She didn't have very many dark ones; she was always making sure I was going to be okay. When she said that, I looked at her—this was just a couple days before she passed away—and I promised her that would never happen.

That's how Rhea's Tower came about at the ranch. Whenever Rhea came to Aspen, she'd always look at the sky for shooting stars. That was what she loved so much about Colorado because in Chicago, she couldn't see the stars because of the night lights. We would look for shooting stars, and we'd wander about, saying, "Oh, did you see one? Did you see one?" Rhea's Tower is the highest place on the ranch. It's the closest point to the stars. We named it Rhea's Tower so everyone would always remember her spirit and her love of life and her appreciation of the time we have here, because no one ever knows how long that will be.

(Courtesy of authors, excerpt from *You Go Girl!*)

"I don't think you choose this career. I think it chooses you."

— *Andrea Jaeger*

Samatha Imus—cancer survivor
Twenty-six years old—Ribera, New Mexico
Ranch coordinator, The Imus Ranch

The Imus Ranch is an authentic working cattle ranch. It was conceived and designed with the sole purpose of providing the experience of the great American cowboy to children suffering from cancer or serious blood disorders, and children who have lost brothers and sisters to Sudden Infant Death Syndrome.

Our objective is to give them a sense of achievement, responsibility, and self-esteem, and to instill pride and restore their dignity as they become aware of just how much they are able to accomplish. Many have become convinced that because they are sick, they are not normal. At The Imus Ranch, they quickly discover that they can do anything any other kid can do, and that there is life after treatment. We have an oncologist, a registered nurse, and two child life specialists with us every session. This will be our fourth summer.

The ranch is a magnificent facility with nearly 4,000 acres and a western town that rivals any movie set in Hollywood. All the kids become part of the extended family, living together in a 14,000 square foot adobe hacienda. The kids spend a week at the ranch. Because this is a real working ranch, children have either completed their treatment or are on maintenance. They're up at six in the morning, and they're basically regular ranch hands. It's all part of their next step of recovery.

The children spend their days doing chores side by side with ranch wranglers. They round up cattle, herd and feed the sheep, the buffalo, the chickens, goats, and donkeys. They learn to care for their own horse. They take part in the dawn to dusk rhythms of a western ranch while developing a bond with animals, which will last a lifetime. When children suffering from these frightening diseases are exposed to the programs that we offer at The Imus Ranch, it often contributes to their healing and recovery.

We operate in the summer from the end of June to the end of August. We have eight sessions of ten kids, ages eleven to seventeen, who come for nine days of the summer, with a two-day break between each session.

We had a girl who was very, very sick when she was little. She had to have both hips replaced, had been on mega steroids her whole life, and she had a heart condition. She had never ridden a horse before, so we found her a sidesaddle and she was able to ride like any other kid. Her grin stretched from ear to ear. She's a remarkable young lady. She actually ended up working at the ranch this summer. She'd been out here as a ranch hand for a couple of years, and then we hired her this summer. So that's pretty incredible.

We had a boy who had every illness in the world; I can't even remember all of them. I know that he had cancer in his heart, his lungs, his liver, in basically everything. As a result of radiation and chemo, he had become deaf, and yet he's one of the most incredible kids I've ever met. He's the most outgoing young person, and he reads lips. He's almost 100 percent deaf but he lip-reads at 100 percent, so you wouldn't even know he's deaf. He's amazing, and everyone is drawn to him.

The Imus Ranch is run completely on donations, so there is no charge. In addition, Don Imus, the founder, gives to the ranch and spreads the word via his national radio and TV show. We're a non-profit organization. Anyone who wants to come to the ranch can call me, but the final decision is up to their medical professionals. The children's own oncologists and nurses know if they are through treatment and are healthy enough to come out. It's a great adventure.

Maija Bradshaw
Thirty-two years old—Lake Rosseam, Ontario, Canada
Executive director, Camp Oochigeas

Camp Oochigeas is a camp for children who have cancer. As one camper said, "At Camp Oochigeas, no one really pays attention to the fact that you have cancer because everyone does." The name is taken from the legend of Princess Oochigeas, a young Canadian-Indian girl who overcame physical hardships through courage and bravery.

The camp is a fantastic place that started back in 1984. That first summer we had thirty kids, and it ran for only five days. The summer of 2003 is our twentieth year and we'll have 200 kids, ages six to seventeen, and it will run for six weeks.

It's a pretty amazing place; we are what people call the *social cure* for cancer. There is a lot we can do medically for cancer, but there are many hidden things, like self-esteem and self-confidence, that also get hurt by cancer. Those are what we try to help kids deal with. We try to be honest, and we give them two weeks of being a kid again, doing things they would normally do.

A lot of these children know more about drug names and about cancer treatment than we adults do. Camp gives them an opportunity to let them forget they've got cancer and be a regular kid for awhile. Cancer takes away their childhood, so we give it back to them with a sense of carefree freedom and no responsibility.

This is the only camping facility in Ontario that offers chemotherapy treatment on-site for our kids so they don't need to go to a hospital to get their therapy. They can do it right on the property. We have doctors and nurses from The Hospital for Sick Children in Toronto who make it happen. They come here and give these kids the best two weeks of their year. The kids come away stronger, physically, mentally, and emotionally. It's unbelievable how much energy we see.

We're like a traditional camp, with swimming, canoeing, kayaking, and arts and crafts, almost anything under the sun. All of our staff are volunteers, which makes camp a really special place. We have 230 people who come from many different walks of life. They are teachers, lawyers, accountants, and they volunteer for one or two weeks, offering their skills and talents to create this incredibly dynamic place.

We have all the regular camp activities, and then there is the occasional chocolate pudding fight, the big water slide, the polar bear dip, tubing on a giant inflatable banana, the party barge, and all those things that only happen at camp. Attending Camp Oochigeas is like lifting the blinds and letting the sunshine in. It's amazing.

Chapter Four
Women's Choice

Some of the best news in cancer research applies to women's breast cancer. The latest advances will increase the odds of detecting and treating breast cancer sooner and surviving it longer. Much of the information focuses on making diagnosis and treatment more effective, less invasive (a major key), and with fewer side effects.

The newest tools may include:

1. MRI—Magnetic Resonance Imaging helps find "hidden" breast cancer.
2. Ductoscopy—A tiny camera inserted through the nipple.
3. Ductal Lavage—Exploration of tiny milk ducts with a minuscule catheter.
4. Lymphoseek—New imaging agent to single out "sentinel lymph nodes."
5. PET scan—Position Emission Tomography scanning will eventually outperform a mammogram.
6. Brachytherapy—Implanting tiny "seeds" of radiation twice daily for a week instead of radiation treatments every day for six or more weeks.
7. Icon—A new drug that targets metastic breast cancer that is resistant to chemotherapy and hormone therapy.

Anne Wallace, M.D., F.A.C.S.

Forty-one years old—La Jolla, California
Surgical oncologist and plastic surgeon, UCSD's Moores Cancer Center

We have to change our thought process. We have to start thinking "outside the breast." We have to start finding cancer not only when it's small, but also when it is going to be biologically important, and then figure out why.

There are a few cancers that are lethal from the get-go, for instance pancreatic cancer or esophageal cancer. However, breast cancer and prostate cancer are similar in that many of these cancers would never kill anyone even if they were never treated. At this point, though, we just don't know which are which.

Right now, the diagnosis of breast cancer is far from a death sentence, and even if you have breast cancer, we can keep you alive for many, many years with lots of different classes of drugs. If one drug doesn't work, we have another one we can try. You could write a book, a very big book, just on medical therapy for breast cancer.

I don't think we'll have a cure for breast cancer in five years. I'm hoping to see it in my lifetime, but I doubt that if you're diagnosed with breast cancer in five years you'll be able to say, "I don't need to worry about this, I'm cured." We are just not that far along.

In the mid-90s, we didn't know anything about prevention of breast cancer. Now, however, we are beginning to understand genes and how they lead to cancer. Soon we'll be able to manipulate those genes. However, the big thing we have to be on the lookout for is that we don't know the consequences of manipulating genes, and that may lead to other disease processes.

We're a little way from this, but we're getting closer every day. We merely need to keep plugging along at the molecular level until we finally understand it. But, I don't think it will happen tomorrow.

The good news is that we're doing more and more breast conservation, which means we don't have to remove the breast. However, we have found that since the year 2000, increasing numbers of younger women have elected to have their breast taken off, and yet, during this same time period, women between the ages of sixty and seventy-five have been devastated by losing theirs. I'm not sure if this is because of their generation; perhaps older women place more significance in their breasts as a part of their self-image, but I'm trying to figure it out.

Another advancement is that reconstruction options are getting increasingly more elaborate. We are trying very hard to get women to look good to the naked eye, not just be good looking in clothes.

"It's amazing how many women and girls don't know very much about their breasts. It's very, very important that we educate our daughters and our sisters about that part of the anatomy."

— *Joy Shephard—breast cancer,*
survivor of the 9/11 World Trade
Center tragedy

David Hodgens, M.D.

Fifty-eight years old—La Jolla, California
Medical Director of Radiation Oncology, Scripps Memorial Hospital

A woman's sense of herself is to a great degree tied to her feminine appearance. Obviously, a large part of that is her breasts. That's true from the youngest women we see in their teens and their twenties, to the older women. Across the board it's an important part of their own view of themselves.

Dr. Charlie Campbell was one of the pioneers here at Scripps for doing what we call breast conservation. In other words, pushing the surgeons to do less breast surgery, and instead do a lumpectomy, followed by radiation. This has become the most common way of treating early breast cancer. Frankly, the motivation has been twofold. One of the principle reasons has been that women don't want to lose their breasts. They don't want to deal with that psychological effect. The second major motivation for it has been the big studies that have proven lumpectomy and radiation are just as effective as mastectomy in curing breast cancer, and in preventing the recurrence of breast cancer.

We say, "Look, you don't have to lose your breasts. You can have a lumpectomy; part of the tumor will be taken out, along with some breast tissue around it. Then we can give radiation to your breasts." The cosmetic effect of that is usually far more satisfactory to most women than losing their breasts by having a mastectomy.

It's sometimes not perfect, but there are many women we've treated over the years who you can't determine which side we've treated. What was interesting to me about it, though, was that I could talk to a thirty-five-year-old woman during one consultation and she would say, "It doesn't really matter to me whether I have a lumpectomy or a mastectomy, so I'll think about it." And that woman might opt for a mastectomy. Then I'd have a seventy-five-year-old woman who would say, "There's no way anybody's going to take my breasts off." I learned that you have to let each woman put her own value on her breasts and you can't necessarily infer that just because a woman is older, she's going to be more amenable to a mastectomy as opposed to a younger woman. I saw women making decisions that, to me, were inconsistent with their age or station in life. But it taught me something. It taught me that you present the options and let the patient and her family members make the decision.

"Mammography is not the final answer to the early detection of breast cancer, but it's the best tool we have now."

— *Dr. Andrew von Eschenbach,*
Director of the National Cancer
Institute

Stephen H. Friend, M.D., Ph.D.

Forty-nine years old—West Point, Pennsylvania
Vice President, Basic Research, Merck & Co., Inc.

The work I'm most familiar with is in breast cancer, where right now 80 percent of the patients are given chemotherapy when they have early stage disease, to try to keep them from getting metastatic disease. We will soon be able to identify whether they even need the treatment. That is, four out of every five patients will have a disease that actually does not need treatment.

The reason they survived is not that the treatment did anything. And that's something pretty frightening. So many patients say, "I'm so glad I went through all that because at least I didn't get the tumor." Well, what would happen if the reality was that they didn't need it in the first place? The treatment did not allow them to survive. They did it themselves.

"Most people who get breast cancer survive it. That is an important message."

> — *Dr. Nancy Davidson,*
> *Director of the Breast Cancer Research*
> *program at The Johns Hopkins*
> *Oncology Center*

Joy Shephard—breast cancer

Sixty-three years old—Escondido, California
Retired school teacher, financial planner, and 9/11 World Trade Center survivor

I was positive it was just a false alarm. The doctor assured me I only had a one out of four chance of cancer. But he needed to have a biopsy just to make sure. So when he called me the next day and told me I had breast cancer, I was in shock that this was happening to me.

I had a single mastectomy. Although the cancer hadn't spread to the lymph nodes, the surgery and complications from it almost killed me. First I had necrotic tissue, which was expanding. Then I had to go in for more surgery. I was allergic to the anesthetic or something they gave me in the hospital, and I went through a period where I couldn't breathe and I couldn't swallow. Then after the second surgery, I had a terrible infection. I had four different bacteria raging through my body at the same time.

I thought I was having a hot flash. My husband and my mother took my temperature and it was 103.5. So they called the Doctor's Exchange and were told, "Keep her cool all night long and bring her to emergency in the morning."

The next day this Japanese infectious disease specialist came to the hospital and I had a third surgery. Oh, boy, that was something. They had to wash all that infection out, just scrape and scrape and scrape. I was awake during it all, scrape and scrape and scrape and irrigate and irrigate and irrigate, and all this stuff kept coming out. They left the wound open and I was put on IVs for four weeks.

On the fourth day, after the complications, I went home from the hospital. I had nurses coming to the house around the clock. My mother stayed with me for four and a half months; my husband was in the midst of selling his business and was under terrible stress during that time. My mother lived with us until I got back on my feet. The cancer was finished; they got it in the early stages and it was finished. That's the way I look at it.

Our refrigerator was filled with plastic IV stuff filled with antibiotics, and I was on a regimen of very strong pills. I was a high school mathematics teacher so I made a matrix to figure out when to take the medicine, which to take, and when not to take it. The nurses were coming every four hours. My dear mother would get up and answer the door, my angel. They would clean the wound and change my bandages, and I had a special pail that was sealed that they threw everything into, including the needles. That was really something. I didn't think I would ever get over it. But the prayers and the support and love of family and friends really kept me upbeat.

I don't know what the key is, but I had a positive attitude. I really believe in the power of prayer, which I think pulled me through. I wasn't supposed to make it; I really wasn't. I was just there. I felt like a piece of limp meat. I remember mother getting me up to try to walk. After three weeks, they put me on a portable IV, which was attached to my body, like this big suitcase. Just what I needed. My mother said, "This is going to get you out of the house and we're going to go shopping." I could barely walk. Oh, she was fabulous.

She took me over to J.C. Penney's to buy me a house dress so I could get out of my nightgown and my bathrobe. So there I was in my nightgown and bathrobe, and my IV and slippers, going into J.C. Penney's. My mother just told everybody we passed, "She had surgery and we're going shopping." She bought me a cute little white and blue house dress that buttoned down the front so I could wear the IV and be dressed. She was amazing.

As soon as I was able to get up—I mean, I could barely walk—we went to Costco. Mother wanted to treat me to lunch but I couldn't swallow very well, so I had one of those soft serve ice creams. It did taste good, but I could only eat half of it. Then I had to hang onto the Costco shopping cart for dear life. My mother said, "I think she's getting a little tired," so we went home. This turned out to be a Friday thing. Every Friday, my sister, my mother, and my sister's friend and I would go to the shopping mall and go for a little walk and maybe a little bit of lunch and then come home. I think getting out helped.

Cancer was the first of my two life-threatening experiences. After retiring from teaching, I began a new career as a financial planner, and I went to New York City for training. I'm not sure if my coping with breast cancer helped me cope with my experience in the World Trade Center on 9/11, but perhaps it did prepare me to deal with the unknown.

I was on the 61st floor of Tower Two in the World Trade Center on the morning of September 11, 2001. After the first explosion, I was positive I saw the tail of a huge airplane in Tower One, a jumbo jet, and I knew something terrible had happened.

One of the managers came out to usher us back to the offices, but I braced myself at the door, looked up at him, and said, "You can't do this. I'm going to walk down the stairs. If everything's all right, I'll come back up."

I started down the stairwell and as I approached the 44th floor, I heard a speaker, another message. But I couldn't understand it in the stairwell, so I stepped out into the hallway, by the elevator, to hear more clearly. The announcement said, "Tower Two is secure. Go back to your offices."

In the meantime, the elevator filled with people and they were holding the door open for me. They said, "Come on, we're going up." Again I hesitated. Should I or shouldn't I? I started to step with my right foot into the elevator, I remember that. Then I backed out, held the door open, and said, "You guys, I can't do this. I'm sorry. I'm going to walk down the stairs."

I was only about five or six steps into the stairwell when the plane hit our building. I knew exactly what it was. I felt the terror because almost immediately I could smell the jet fuel and see the smoke. The stairwell filled up with heat and debris. Straight ahead of me, I could see a large crack in the wall. I could see daylight through it. I knew something terrible had happened. And I also knew something terrible had happened to that elevator.

Luckily, I had worn flats that day, so I was jumping up and down in the stairwell. The building went forward, the stairs came back, and then it shook from side to side. Women screamed all around me and were knocked down under the stairs; they had worn high heels. I don't know why I was so calm. Something came over me; maybe it was the teacher in me. I'd taught high school math for many years and had been through many disaster training exercises. I shouted, "I'm from California. This is like a little earthquake. We get them all the time." And I shook my head as if to say, don't worry. They looked up at me like I was some kind of a nut.

The woman sitting down in front of me said, "I can't get up." I told her, "You're going to have to get up, honey. You've got to get up. There'll be a real disaster if you don't get up. You can do it." I sounded like my mother, with this can-do attitude. I grabbed her hand and she looked up at me. But she got up. I said, "We're going to do this together; we're going to put one foot in front of the other until we get down to the bottom of the stairs."

At that moment, this horrible fear came over me, and I felt like something evil had happened. I really, really did. Then I started praying the Lord's Prayer out loud. Then I prayed Hail Mary. I prayed my Guardian Angel prayer. I spoke to my mother's spirit. I realized that evil was happening here. I recited the Twenty-third Psalm over and over again. I made a good act of contrition because I thought this was going to be it for me. I just asked for God's help. We were all praying together, a whole group of us. I didn't know these people; they were complete strangers. We were all praying together and we sang *Amazing Grace* together.

I met a young man named Mike in the stairwell. He asked me like a little boy, "Can I hold your hand?" This was a big strapping athletic guy in his thirties. I thought, Right. He needs to hold the hand of a sixty-two-year-old woman to get down. He was offering to help me, of course, but he turned it around to make it seem like I was helping him.

So here I am, and the stairwell is only wide enough for two people. I'm holding hands with the woman on my left who's at my level. Her friend is in front of us, and I'm holding hands with Mike who is up above me. I'm walking down the stairs like that with my right hand above and left hand below. I'm praying and singing *Amazing Grace* and reciting the Twenty-third Psalm. Everybody's being positive. We moved together so beautifully;

no one panicked. We settled into this rhythm, just winding, praying, and singing. We moved like one giant organism all the way down the stairs.

New York City firemen greeted us at the bottom with flashlights. We were in this very dark black tunnel. One asked me, "Are you okay?" I said, "I'm fine." And then I pointed to the woman whose hand I'd been holding. He could see that she wasn't well, so he put an oxygen mask on her, and he and another firefighter carried her off on a stretcher. That was the last time I saw her. I didn't even know her name.

Those firemen were like centurions, standing there at their posts and directing us with their flashlights. They were motioning us to go to our right and up some stairs. Pretty soon we were on the concourse level. Ahead of us were throngs of people trying to get out through the revolving doors. Mike was still with me and we both had the same idea. We held hands and we ran to the far right door nobody was using, and we made it to the outside.

First, I thought, Oh, I made it. But that was just the beginning. Then all the horror started, absolute utter horror. I began to hear popping sounds. Initially, I didn't know what they could be. Then I realized it was the sound of bodies hitting the sidewalk. A lot of people were falling, parts of people, burned people. It was horrible. Parts of the concrete of the building, the skin of the building, were falling off at the same time. The people all around us on the ground were getting hit and killed. I don't know why we were missed because it was all around us. Isn't that strange? It was all around us.

It was as though I was walking through this tunnel and people were falling around us. I just talked to them and said, "I'm going to respect you. I'm giving you dignity. I'm not going to stare at you. I commend your souls unto the Lord today. You have nothing more to prove on this earth." That's all I could do. It was the most utterly helpless feeling. Yet, we just kept walking straight. We didn't dodge anything. Everything dodged us. It was a very, very surrealistic experience.

My two life threatening experiences were entirely different but in one sense, they were very similar. One took place over a period of months, and the other was packed into one morning. Yet, in a way, the coping was the same—have a strong faith, have a get-up-and-go attitude, and surround yourself with supportive people.

I've been twice blessed. I know our time on earth is finite. None of us knows how, when, or where we will leave. I do know life is precious. Enjoy it.

Nellie B. Connally—breast cancer
Eighty-three years old—Houston, Texas
Widow of former Texas governor John Connally

I was sleeping with my hands up on this bony part of my upper chest, and one little finger was down toward my left breast. I felt something strange. I knew instantly it was cancer, but I didn't want to believe it. This was about twelve years ago. So I didn't do anything about it for a few weeks. I thought it might go away, but I could be wrong. Of course, it didn't go away.

I went to my doctor and he examined me. He said, "We're going to have to have a biopsy. Who is your surgeon?" I said, "Surgeon? I don't have a surgeon." He said, "I'll get you the best one we have here at Methodist Hospital."

So I went to see the doctor and they did a biopsy. My husband John was with me, and when I came out from the biopsy I was in a strange little room with this doctor and he said, "It is malignant, Mrs. Connally. You can either go home and recover from this biopsy, or you can just go right now and have a mastectomy." Of course I yelled, "John!" He came in and I said, "What do you think we ought to do?" John said, "Nellie, if he thinks this has to be done, and all you're going to do is go home, recover, come back, and start again when you're half under sedation right now, I think we ought to go ahead and do it." And we did.

Now, I don't recommend this. I have other recommendations for people. I think that you should have a second opinion, just because it would make you feel better to know for sure. But I went ahead and had a single mastectomy. I didn't have chemo, I had radiation. I got along just fine. I'm knocking on wood right now. I heard John say many times, "I saw my wife defeat cancer." However, you never know whether you have defeated cancer or not. You get through whatever stage you're in, but who knows, I could have it again. I haven't, and it's been twelve years, so I just have my mammograms every year and, so far, I haven't had any problems. I'm as mean as I ever was. I didn't have any reconstruction. I have one breast and the other one is a phony. When you see me you can guess, but you can't touch.

Afterwards, I started working to fight breast cancer with M.D. Anderson and I helped them raise about three million dollars that went to the Nellie B. Connally Breast Cancer Center. And, of course, I still try to raise money for it in various ways.

I was in my room after the surgery and John was there. He was sitting in a chair with his head in his hands. I said, "John, what's the matter?" He said, "Nellie, do you think the stress of our bankruptcy, which we just went through, caused you to have cancer?" I said, "John, if stress causes cancer, I would have had it fifty years ago. I've been under stress ever since I met you."

I know there's a reason I had cancer. What reason? I can't find a good one, but there must be one. Maybe it's because it got me started in helping to fight breast cancer, I don't know.

I drove myself to my radiation treatments. It was just an annoyance. It took no time. It scared me the first time because they put all those lead things all around me, and then they got ready and said, "Now we're going to . . . " and they all left the room. I thought they were rats leaving a sinking ship. But it took no time, and it took care of whatever needed to be taken care of.

I never could understand, "Why me?" But it was me, so what I had to do was go on and get the radiation and recover. And I did. It's like the Kennedy assassination in that I had to go on.

That was a terrible thing. It was unbelievable to be in that car. We were their hosts while they were in Texas. And like a mother with children, I wanted everybody in Texas to like them. In return, I wanted them to be pleased with everybody from our state.

Everything was going along just perfect. I think it was one of the largest turnouts that President Kennedy ever had. We're in Dallas and they're screaming and yelling just to see him, and John had said to me, "Nellie, if they can just see him, they'll vote for him."

We were driving along just utterly joyous over how everything was turning out. I couldn't restrain myself any longer, so I turned around and said,

"Mr. President, you can't say Dallas doesn't love you." He just grinned and kept waving to the crowd.

That was the last thing I said, and the last thing he heard. We turned on Elm Street and were in front of that ugly book depository building. Then there was a shot. It was a loud noise, but I wasn't certain it was a shot because we'd had all sorts of loud noises with motorcycles, bands, and things all around us.

I was in front of Jackie, and John was seated in front of the President. I turned when I heard that noise and looked at the President and his hand flew up to his neck. John heard the noise and knew it was a shot. He turned to his right to look at the President but couldn't see him. Then he turned to his left, doing all this very rapidly. I think he may have gotten a view of him and then he muttered painfully, "No, no, no." He knew then that he had been shot.

As he was turning back, the second shot hit John and went through his chest. He was covered with blood. I reached over to pull him down in my lap to get him out of the line of fire. The doctors told us later, that by pulling him down and getting his hand over his breast somehow, we closed a wound they call a sucking wound. On the battlefield, they stuff shirts in that type of wound, they stuff anything in; because if you don't cover the wound, it will suck air in and the person will die.

Without such actions, we never would have made it to the hospital. The shot that hit John was the second shot, but they always say that it was the first shot. They want to say the first shot went through the President and then went through John. And I say, "In that case, that bullet would have to just hang right there in mid-air while John turned to the right and then turned to his left." That was impossible. I had him down when the third shot came. Within six seconds, all three shots were fired. I didn't look back after I pulled John down in my lap.

But when the third shot came, there was matter, blood, and stuff that was part of the President's head that splattered all over the blue interior of the car, and all over us. In my heart, I knew the President was dead. The Secret Service man shouted to the driver, "Pull out of this caravan and get us to the nearest hospital."

I'm the only one left. John is gone, and the President and Mrs. Kennedy are gone. That's just what I've got, and I've got to get along with what I've got.

Ann Veneman—ductal carcinoma in situ (DCIS)
Fifty-three years old—Washington, D.C.
U.S. Secretary of Agriculture

I had a lumpectomy to remove a ductal carcinoma in situ (DCIS), which is probably the least invasive of all breast cancers. It's just in the cell— there's no lump—it's the most treatable form of cancer. It was detected in a routine mammogram, which is the only way it is discovered, and I immediately had a biopsy.

When I was first told I needed a biopsy, I wasn't concerned. There was no history of cancer in my family, and I was convinced it was going to be negative. Even after the biopsy, I was certain it was going to be negative. When I got the results, I was shocked.

I had a couple of days where I thought, What am I going to do? But then I went full-steam ahead, thinking, I've got to get second opinions. I've got to find the right doctors. I'm going to call the National Cancer Institute. I was determined to get every bit of information I could, so I also called my friend, Nancy Goodman Brinker, the U.S. Ambassador to Hungary, who founded the Susan G. Komen Breast Cancer Foundation.

Of course, I didn't want to miss any work. The only day I did was when I had my lumpectomy. The most important thing was staying busy and staying focused on my regular daily obligations and responsibilities. I sent a letter to friends and colleagues about my cancer. Since I was not able to travel because I was going for radiation everyday, I wanted them to understand why. In my position, I thought it was important to make it public. As it turned out, the week I was going to do this, President Bush was holding a cancer event in the White House, and he announced it, which was quite unusual.

One of the significant things that came out of all this is public awareness. The morning after President Bush made his announcement, I was on the TV show *Good Morning America.* I talked a lot about the importance of screenings, such as PSA tests, colonoscopies, and mammograms.

I received so many letters and cards from people giving me good wishes and saying they were praying for me. Many shared their own stories. In addition, some told me that because of what happened to me, they were going to make an appointment for their mammogram.

One day, I was coming back from a meeting in my department and I ran into a friend of mine from Kansas, who was in town. I've known her for a long time, and while we were chatting, she said, "I have a friend back home who credits you with saving her life. A lot of women listened to what you had to say about screening and mammograms. My friend was one, and through a mammogram her cancer was detected early and she was able to be treated." That was amazing. I mean, many women said they went to get mammograms because they heard my message, but when my friend credits me with saving a life, I was like, wow! Instantly, it took all the cares of the day away from me.

I think life works in mysterious ways, and God just does certain things. The day I found out my biopsy results, my sister had flown in on the red-eye from California to take her daughter to college in Delaware. They were staying with me for a couple days and were at my house when I got the news. My sister just changed her schedule and stayed for another week. We went together to get all the second opinions. I think that's the way God had it planned.

Excerpts from President George W. Bush's speech on September 18, 2002, when he announced a budget increase of $629 million for funding cancer research:

Last month, Secretary of Agriculture Ann Veneman learned she had breast cancer. This is one of the toughest challenges any family will face, including the White House family . . . I'm proud of the example she sets for many women to understand the need to get a mammogram; the need to take care of yourself; the need to screen early; the need to understand that we can stop cancer in its tracks if we all make wise moves. And so, Ann, thank you for your courage and your example.

Suzyn Waldman—breast cancer

Forty-three years old—Croton-on-the-Hudson, New York
New York Yankees television announcer

Your first instinct when you find you have breast cancer is to say, "All right, get it out of me, tell me what I need to do to get on with my life." That's something that you just do. But how do you get on with your life? I don't think I had a choice. You can either go on or you can give up and die, in this case, literally. When given the choice, people will always look at this and say, "Okay, what do I do to go on?"

My first thought was not to tell anybody, but obviously, I had to. Then I found out that people wanted me to go away because I had breast cancer. Everyone was very nice, but it was almost like I was starting over in sports broadcasting. It was, "Yes, dear. When you get better, come back and we'll talk about it."

I was diagnosed three weeks before spring training. That was the first year I was going to have a full-time job as a New York Yankees announcer. I'd worked fifteen years for that. I thought to myself, I can't go away and come back when I'm better. Somebody else will be sitting in my seat.

There's a great saying: "You can't control the wind, but you can control your sails." I thought of that a lot because breast cancer was nothing I had asked for. I had no control over it; but I had control of my sails. But what I discovered was people didn't want me around because I was sick. I didn't feel sick, I didn't look sick, but I was sick. And something else kicked in. I wasn't going to let it beat me. I continued to work. I probably shouldn't have, but I did. It kept me going. It kept me alive.

I remember calling George Steinbrenner on the phone when they were futzing around with my contract. I said, "George, it's Suzyn. Are you not going to give me this job because I have breast cancer?" Just like that. And he said, "What the hell are you talking about?"

I fired my first oncologist because he wouldn't let me go to spring training. I said to the hospital, "You better find me somebody because I'm going to spring training and unless you want me to die, you'd better find a way to do this." They sent me to a supposedly overaggressive female doctor. She was just great with me. She said, "We'll work it out. We'll do this because quality of life is very important when you're fighting breast cancer."

I missed very few games. I missed the day I had chemo, once every three weeks for six months, and I missed the day after because I was so sick. Other than that, I gave myself shots on the plane. The Yankees were awesome. I mean it came out of nowhere. I never would have expected this, but George and the trainers set up doctors for me all over the country, wherever we were, so that I could have my blood tests every few days to make sure I wasn't going to die. I had Neupogen shots to keep my white blood cell count up. They were in every clubhouse in the American League, wherever we were, just in case I needed them. It was amazing.

I found such a network of people who I thought I had only covered professionally and who I had merely stuck a microphone in their face. The guys on the Yankees were great. I traveled with the team; if I started getting nauseous, all of a sudden I'd turn around and there would be some player standing next to me with a club soda. It was incredible. I never said a word. I lost my hair, my eyebrows, my eyelashes, everything. I wore a wig and makeup on television.

I received hundreds and hundreds of letters during that time. I got one from a woman who had stage four breast cancer. This was in 1996. She said, "I just want to thank you because my husband brought home two tickets to the World Series to see my team, the Yankees, and I wouldn't go because I had no hair and I had a crisis. If it hadn't been for you, I would have missed my team winning the World Series because I was saying, 'I can't go, I can't go.' Then I turned on the television and there you were. I looked at the screen and I said if she can do it, I can do it. I put a scarf on my head and I went and saw the Yankees win."

There's so much that goes with being a breast cancer survivor because there's no cure, so it's in the back of your mind every day. It has been ten years and every time I get an ache I think, Oh God, it's back. It doesn't go away. But you learn to live with it and you learn to help other people. It begets other things.

When Darryl Strawberry was diagnosed with cancer, I was there for Darryl. Darryl was there for Joe Torre. Joe was there for you, Charlie. It just keeps going. You can control what you do with it. You're supposed to give something back in this life. Cancer isn't what I would have chosen, and I'm sure it isn't what Joe Torre would have chosen either, but you deal with it.

(Courtesy of the authors, excerpts from *That's Outside My Boat*)

"Our journey is always more fulfilling when we share it with others."

— *Kim Doren,*
co-author

Name withheld by request

Shares her experience with her ninety-four-year-old mother
who is recovering from breast cancer

My mother was ninety-two when she found the lump in her breast. Her doctor had taken the position that women don't have to have mammograms every year after a certain age because the likelihood of breast cancer after age eighty was so remote. However, we learned this is not actually true.

After an examination and biopsy, her doctor took me aside and told me she had breast cancer. He said she had the choice of a mastectomy, a lumpectomy, chemotherapy, radiation, or nothing. I decided not to tell my mother she had cancer because all she would do was worry about it, and I knew she would say to me, "You know more about this than I do. You make the decision."

I did it to protect her but the doctors kept saying I had to tell her. I thought, Why? My mother's sister had breast cancer in the 1950s, and she had a radical mastectomy and suffered greatly. That was my mother's idea of cancer and I didn't want to put that image in her head. She loves her life, and I didn't want her to live everyday fearing death; I wanted her to continue loving her life.

I did a lot of research on what was the best option given her age and situation, and what happened next is a great story of intervention from God. I felt so overwhelmed having to make this decision myself that I kept praying I would be given a sign because I just didn't know what to do. One of my relatives kept saying to do nothing; at her age, it wasn't worth putting her through the discomfort. That was the prevailing opinion. Yet, having done the research, I was inclined to select the lumpectomy and nothing else because I was afraid of what chemo or radiation would do to her.

I prayed about it really hard and in the midst of my prayers, my brother was taking her to the doctor when she tripped and fell on the pavement, broke her glasses, and cut open her face and hand. This accident actually propelled us into a situation that took the decision right out of my hands. It was almost as if God said, "Okay, you need me to do this, and I'm really sorry for the fact that your mother had to go through the fall and her stitches, but here is what you need to do."

As a result of the accident, mother had congestive heart failure, and during her follow-up examination I told the doctor about the lump. Afterward, he told me there was no choice but to have the lump taken care of immediately, and that decided it.

I found a wonderful surgeon who treated my mother with great respect. I told her they needed to remove the lump and that in order for her not to have other ones, she needed treatment. My excuse for the radiation was to prevent additional lumps from developing, which was true. I always called it a lump.

We did a lumpectomy and she had forty-three radiation treatments. She never missed a meal, and never took a nap. It didn't slow her down one bit. She did beautifully. I went to see her after surgery, and when the doctor said, "You can go in now," I said, "I'm not sure I can." He replied, "I'll go with you, she's fine." I entered the recovery room and peeked around the curtain and she said, "Where did you put my earrings?" At that point, I thought, I'm such a weenie. I have a ninety-two-year-old mother who is such a source of strength. How blessed am I?

I think deep down inside she probably knew it was cancer but she had a really positive attitude about it. She even baked cakes to take to the radiologist. Fear will kill you. It's very disabling to people. It was hard enough for me to have that fear; I didn't want her to have it, too.

She's great now. She just passed her eighteen-month test and when she goes for her two-year follow-up they are going to put her on an annual checkup. The largest incidence of cancer returning is in the first two years. Of course, her next goal is five years. My goal is for her to live to at least age 110.

I was never aware of how strong my mother was because I always thought my dad was the strong one in the family. When my father died at age eighty-eight, I really began to realize how strong my mother actually was. The wisdom of age is a beautiful thing, and the way she was able to accept and deal with my father's passing was unbelievable.

When they interview people who have lived at least 100 years, they find that one of the keys to living that long is how they deal with grief. My mother taught me a lot, and she continues to teach me everyday. She loves life; she loves everybody. She doesn't have a critical bone in her body. She's a great example to me.

Denise Connolly—breast cancer at age twenty-six, and again at age thirty-one

Thirty-eight years old—Ft. Thomas, Kentucky
Housewife, mother, and cancer counselor

I was diagnosed with breast cancer when I was twenty-six years old. I had been married for just six months and we were moving from California to northern Kentucky. They discovered the tumor during a routine physical for my teaching job.

I had always been very lumpy but because I was so young, I had never had a mammogram. Well, I had one and they found a two-and-a-half centimeter tumor. It was malignant. First, I had chemotherapy, then a double mastectomy, followed by reconstruction and more rounds of chemo. It all went reasonably well and we completed our move to Kentucky. Everything was going just fine.

Four years later I had our first child and right away I got pregnant again. About four and a half months into the second pregnancy, I noticed a very small lump on one of my reconstructed breasts. It looked like a mosquito bite, and it was in the same exact spot, same breast as the original tumor, between my skin and the implant. It was cancerous.

I began to panic. Everyone around me had this strange look on their face, like I'm supposed to die. The doctors determined that I had stage four cancer, and being four-and-a-half months pregnant, they thought I should have an abortion. Upon hearing this, my husband left the room and threw up. I emphatically said, "No."

I immediately called my original oncologist in California and he said, "Get on the next plane," which I literally did. I was immediately admitted to Scripps Hospital. That night they kept an operating room open and the pathologist on duty. They did a lumpectomy while I was awake because you can't be given anesthesia when you're pregnant.

The pathologist told me he didn't know what the tumor was growing in. It was just sort of a free floater that wasn't attached to anything. I had this strange malignant tumor, so we treated it like stage four cancer.

We decided to induce pregnancy a month early, thinking my baby would be just fine. However, her lungs weren't fully developed and she was on the critical list for sixteen days. Fortunately, she pulled through with flying colors.

We started the stage four cancer treatments, three rounds of chemo followed by a double bone marrow transplant using my own stem cells. Next, I had seven weeks of radiation followed by three more rounds of Paxil chemotherapy. I'm a very happy, optimistic person and I always thought that as long as I know I have a chance, I'll handle it. Just give me a chance to survive and I'll do it.

I kept a notebook when I was going through all my treatments and at the end of each day, I would rejoice over crossing off another day. Since this was the second time I had cancer, I would also write, "You're going to feel better today," or "Your hair will start to grow properly about now."

Also, because it was stage four cancer, I really didn't know what the outcome would be. So I often wrote to my children, knowing that the odds were against me being around in their future. I would write how much I loved them, what my hopes and dreams were for them, and what I saw them doing with their lives. My girls are now seven and nine years old. I haven't shown them the notebook yet, but I will someday. And that will be a very special time.

I finished all my treatments in May of 1996, more than seven years ago. Both our daughters are doing well, and I'm as clean as a whistle. My progress has been terrific, and I think I'm going to make it. After all, my doctor tells me I have the strongest will to live that he has ever known. He refers to me as his "tough broad."

"As I look back, I was so young. I was twenty-six and just married when I had my double mastectomy. I don't recall any loss of my sex drive. Age probably had a lot to do with it, and things are still okay, thus far."

— *Denise Connolly*

Mary Allan—breast cancer, tumor in pelvis, osteoarthritis
Sixty-three years old—La Jolla, California
Community volunteer and horse jumper

It is terrifying when you're first diagnosed with cancer. You wake up in the morning with a sick stomach and just think, Oh, my gosh, and your heart is all squeezed and you feel like, What's wrong? Then you remember what's wrong. And you say, "How can I get through this?" But familiarity breeds contempt. I have contempt for my cancer. I keep telling it, "I'm going to get you."

I was first diagnosed fourteen years ago with breast cancer and thought I was going to die. My father died from cancer. However, after a mastectomy, I was cancer-free for ten years. Then my cancer returned.

I was really mad. I was in total denial. I was telling myself, "I don't have cancer again. Forget it. They're wrong." Then I looked at my x-rays and thought, Maybe they're not wrong. I was really feisty about it. I was sulking. But I'm a fighter, I really am. I'm not one to lay down my sword.

The third time I thought, Okay, here we go again. Just acceptance. This is something I'm going to be fighting; sort of chronic cancer. It's controllable, but they don't know if it's going to be curable in my lifetime.

In a strange way, it's almost a gift because I enjoy life so much more now. The love and support I've had from my family and friends has been incredible. My cancer has been a kind of skewed gift.

This is going to sound really dumb, but I feel it's my mission to show women that this is something you don't have to be terrified of. It's something you can do. You can face it and have a good life. It's doable. That's my passion—to show that this is not the end of your life, and that you just have to get through it. You do the best you can, you do what you have to do, and then you go on.

I cope by not accepting any other solution other than that I'm going to be okay. I'm doing really well and my numbers have come down. I'm close to being done with my third treatment. I feel good. I think a positive attitude is very important in your cure, and in your results. I'm just a positive, stubborn person.

I'm back on track again. I go out. I don't turn down any invitations; I do everything I can. If I'm going to go out in the evening, I'll take a nap. That's all it really takes, and I go out and have a good time.

"My situation, as bad as it is, has made me view life in a different way. That work is work—not life. That I should not be thinking, I'll do that one day, but to do things now and not wait. To appreciate the people in my life; to appreciate everything as much as possible. To make sure I have as few regrets as possible."

— *Adriana Jenkins—aggressive breast cancer, doctors give her only a 40 percent chance of remaining cancer-free over the next five years*

Minerva Kunsel—ovarian cancer and breast cancer
Eighty-two years old—La Jolla, California
Housewife, mother, grandmother, and widow

During my recovery from ovarian cancer in my mid-forties, I collected sympathy and tender loving care from my friends like a cheap panhandler. That did help me keep my attitude, but my cancer forced me to change my perspective of time.

I got to the point where I could look at something and say, "I haven't a lot of time, and I don't know how much it is going to cost me in time." It's like money in the bank. Am I going to spend it on this, or am I going to spend it on that? I sorted out my time priorities.

I found I was enjoying simple things, in the moment. It was almost spiritual, like I had been looking through a veil. Before it was fuzzy, and now it was bright Technicolor. Each day was a gift. It was a vivid experience to find I could be in the moment. All of this made my attitude very positive.

My husband and I discovered that funny movies were wonderful. That may have been our trick. We'd rent comedies, three at a time, and we found that laughter really helps. It's good medicine. It always was, and it was especially good medicine during my recovery.

For my ovarian cancer, I had radiation and a kind of chemotherapy they no longer do. Because the cancer had metastasized in both ovaries, they injected the chemotherapy and had me stand on my head for an hour, then on my feet for an hour, then lie down on one side for an hour, and then lie down on my other side. I was swishing the chemo all around to kill any cancer cells that might have escaped during surgery. That, along with the radiation, pretty much took care of it.

However, I was taking an estrogen replacement so, naturally, fourteen years later I got breast cancer. This was awful. Now, I'm really taking my hair down. Ovarian cancer doesn't show. In the long run, it doesn't change your physique very much. But when you lose bosoms, you lose your self-image as an attractive female in a nice body. That was discouraging. I wept for days.

When two of my best friends, who were breast cancer survivors, heard that I was struggling, they brought me a teddy bear with big Band-Aids across the bosoms. When I could laugh at myself, things got much better.

"Aftershock, disbelief, frightened, mortality, introspection, game plan, do it, be thankful each day. These are the emotional jolts I went through before and after my double mastectomy."

— *Ann Williams Jones—breast cancer survivor since 1983*

Isobel "Izzy" Leverant—breast cancer
Fifty-five years old—San Diego, California
Homemaker and mother

A woman I don't know called me today for some radiation information. I told her to expect to be tired and let yourself be tired. Let people around you help, because too often we don't let that happen; we have to do everything ourselves. Give into it.

There's a wonderful deodorant you can use. I mean, it sounds like a stupid thing, but you can use it when you have radiation because it's all natural. You have to wet it to use it, and it looks like a crystal, but I can't remember its name. There are also special creams and soaps. Aloe is also really good. Those are things that you can use during treatment. It helps to use a lot of creams and lotions.

I also told her to schedule her treatment appointments around the same time if possible. This helps you establish a schedule, which becomes a natural part of your day. But most importantly, the two main things are to let the people around you help, and when you're tired, lie down and rest.

"I never had that 'I don't want to get up in the morning' feeling. My son was in eighth grade and my daughter was in tenth. If anything, I was more stoic. I didn't want anything to stop me."

— "Izzy" Leverant

Linda Merkins—breast cancer that metastasized to her bones, liver, and brain during a ten-year period
Fifty-eight years old—La Jolla, California
Wife, mother, and grandmother

There is a loss of the sex drive among women who have breast cancer. Absolutely. At first it may be psychological, you feel non-sexual because a part of you is missing. The sex drive is different for women, anyway. We're not driven by whatever the guys are driven by. I've never been sure what that is; guys are driven by everything.

To be graphic, whether or not you lose a breast, you're going to take drugs and have some kind of chemotherapy program or have your ovaries removed. Once any of those things happen, you are going to have painful consequences. There is nothing left to produce any kind of secretions. It's like the Sahara Desert.

For some women who have had a lumpectomy, there is no interruption of their sex drive, but for a woman who has had any kind of extensive treatment, it's just too debilitating. Physically and physiology-wise it becomes extremely difficult.

"I once went into a bone marrow transplant and a doctor said to me, 'This is ridiculous. All we're doing is buying time.' I thought, Hallelujah. That's what I'm trying to do here. That's the name of the game."

— *Linda Merkins*

Anne Dick—apocrine cancer of the secretory cells of the breast
Fifty-nine years old—La Jolla, California
Community volunteer, wife, and mother

I'd had my first chemo and when I came home, I thought, Well, I guess I'll just wait to get sick. Nothing happened, so I started to fix dinner and pretty soon my husband Chuck came home; I fixed a drink, everything was just fine, and we had a wonderful dinner. I looked at him and said, "I'm really kind of tired, would you mind cleaning up the kitchen?" He replied, "Not at all. I'll be up shortly."

I was sitting on our king-size bed, sobbing, when Chuck came in and asked, "Oh, Annie, what's the matter?" I said, "Oh, Chuck, this chemo and everything isn't going to work. Apocrine is such a rare cancer, they don't know if the treatment will work or not. They don't know anything about what I have." He said, "Wait, wait. Just a minute."

He put on his pajamas, crawled in bed with me, and placed his head right on my thigh. I was sobbing, saying, "This is not going to work. I know it's not going to work." And I looked down at Chuck and there he was, snoring. So I lifted his head and put it on his pillow and said, "Well, screw you. I'll guess I'll just have to take care of myself."

"My doctor told me my breast tissue was actually a sweat gland. I said, 'Keep that a secret because all the guys wouldn't be so fascinated with them if they knew they were only sweat glands.'"

— *Anne Dick*

"One of the first things I did was to share my bad news of breast cancer with everyone as soon as I could. I don't keep things to myself. Suddenly, you're not alone with this great big dark secret."

— *Betsy Carter—breast cancer,*
editor-in-chief of My Generation

"As many as thirty studies have shown that women who exercise at moderate to vigorous levels a minimum of three hours a week can reduce their risk of developing breast cancer by 30 to 40 percent."

— *Dr. Anne McTierman,*
author of Breast Fitness

Chapter Five

Largest Men's Club in America

If you're an American man over fifty years of age, the odds are that eventually you will be diagnosed with prostate cancer. It is simply a part of the aging process.

However, the good news is, prostate cancer is becoming, for the most part, a curable disease. The treatment—surgery and radiation—is becoming increasingly more effective, as is the treatment for advanced prostate cancer.

Yet, if you live long enough, in all probability, you will have a form of prostate cancer. As with all cancers, early detection is crucial.

Patrick C. Walsh, M.D.

Sixty-three years old—Baltimore, Maryland
Director of the Brady Urological Institute at The Johns Hopkins
Medical Institutions

I deal with a different category of patients. To be honest, most of the people I see today already know they have prostate cancer. The thing about men, especially men at a typical prostate cancer age, is that they've been through life. So after a positive biopsy, it's not unusual for a man to say, "You know, Dr. Walsh, I always figured I'd get some kind of cancer. Prostate cancer, as I understand, is one you can cure. Of all the cancers I might have gotten, in this respect, it's not the worst in the world."

I can't say anyone is ever happy to know they have it. But I would say that most men who find out they have prostate cancer are able to accept it, decide what to do about it, and then treat it.

I send a lot of people for radiation, but I don't radiate them. I operate on people. After operations, people have a lack of energy. We give them common sense advice such as, "If you're tired, take a nap." Men can be a little macho, so when they wake up and feel well, they should exercise. If they don't exercise, they're never going to regain their strength. They also have to understand that being tired is normal. I tell them, "You're not tired because the cancer is galloping through your body. You're tired because this is the way your body is reacting to this treatment. You're going to be fine."

John Mendelsohn, M.D.

Sixty-six years old—Houston, Texas
President of the University of Texas, M.D. Anderson Cancer Center

Prostate cancer can be a devastating disease; when it spreads outside the prostate, it can cause pain, it can cause obstruction, it can get into your bones and cause spontaneous fractures.

I think the point that needs to be made here is that prostate cancer is a very strange disease. If every man over age seventy had a biopsy done, well over half would have little bits of cancer in their prostate, which would only be important for maybe 4 percent of all those people. For the rest of them, it's not important.

But if you've learned about it, what do you do then? Knowing that prostate cancer can be very slow growing and that it's a non-clinical problem in the majority of cases in which it exists, presents a tremendous challenge. We need to find a way to do studies on the cancer and discern which of the patients (in whom you detect a little trace of prostate cancer) are in that 4 percent range where you should do something very aggressive, and which ones aren't.

Until we know the answer to that, anybody in their right mind, who knows there's a substantial chance that his cancer could get worse, is going to think very carefully about doing aggressive therapy, even though he may not need it. This is going to be a challenge for all of us to deal with, and we're working on it in the research area.

E. David Crawford, M.D.

Fifty-five years old—Denver, Colorado
Section Head of Urological Oncology at University of Colorado Health Science
Center, chairman of Prostate Cancer Education Council

Because prostate cancer is so common and is the second leading cause of men's death, we have three strategies. One is to prevent it. Two is to find it early, treat it and cure it. And three is to find some way to cure the disease in its advanced stages.

We've made strides in all those areas, but the one that provides the most immediate gratification is the early detection. We're involved in a number of studies to prevent prostate cancer. But even if we knew how to prevent it today, it would be years before we would see any impact on the death rate from the disease.

We tailor treatment to the patient. We have a multi-disciplinarian team that consists of urologists, medical oncologists, and radiation oncologists. We evaluate all the patients, and probably half will have surgery, 40 percent will have radiation, and 10 percent will continue to be observed. We tend to recommend surgery on the younger men who have cancer confined in their prostate.

As men live longer, there is going to be more prostate cancer. For that reason, I think it's a disease where we can really help people. But we still have a long way to go. We're finding and probably treating men who don't need to be treated, and we're missing men who need to be treated. There is still a lot to learn.

Gerald Wahman, M.D.

Sixty-six years old—Fort Smith, Arkansas
Senior urologist, Sparks Medical Plaza

There are several answers to the question: What should a patient expect after radiation or surgery, or other treatment? Let's talk about surgery first. Aside from getting over a major surgical procedure, like anything that involves a major abdominal incision, you have fatigue and tiredness. If your blood count's a little low and you did not receive a transfusion, it takes awhile to rebuild your blood count.

The major complications of surgery are sexual impotence, which you try to avoid by doing what is called a nerve-sparing radical prostatectomy. Dr. Patrick Walsh at Johns Hopkins described that procedure.

Many patients who have prostate cancer already have some relative impotence before the surgery. There are different ways of dealing with the impotence should that occur. Viagra sometimes works. There's what's called self-injection therapy, a vacuum device for erections, or a penile prosthesis.

The other major complication of surgery is incontinence, which is the loss of urinary control, and it can vary in degree. Some people have just a very slight amount, a drop or two of urine if they cough hard or sneeze unexpectedly, others have to wear pads because of leakage that's significant. People just sort of learn to live with the minor leakage in one way or another.

Most people are ingenious enough that they adopt whatever is necessary. If they have a cold and they're coughing, they may wear some pads, but for the most part, during their daily activities, they don't leak. If there's a lot of leakage, then there's a urinary sphincter that can be implanted, which usually takes care of the problem. That's just an overview of surgery. If we are going to do surgery and anticipate the need for transfusion, we like to have people donate their own blood to receive it back. That's called autologous transfusion.

Then there's brachytherapy, little seeds that are implanted into the prostate tissue. They give high radiation energy, but it travels a very short distance. There are fairly rigid criteria in terms of the Gleason score and the extent of disease demonstrated in the prosthetic biopsies to use brachytherapy alone. Most of the patients who have brachytherapy alone do pretty well post-operatively and are able to resume reasonable normal activity fairly quickly. But an occasional patient will have difficulty with urinary hesitancy or retention. If they have difficulty emptying, there are medications, such as Flomax, which is an alpha-one blocker that helps relax the bladder and can facilitate voiding.

Some patients have to learn to do intermittent catheterization for a period of time, or wear a catheter. We don't really like to do any surgical intervention on the brachytherapy patients for at least six months because if you go in and do the trans-urethral resection of the prostate and remove the seeds, you've lost the effect of the seeds. With the I-125 isotope that we commonly use, the radiation effect is pretty well dissipated by six months. We like to avoid surgery until that period of time.

Some patients will have rectal problems, usually that's a later development. A year to a year-and-a-half post-brachytherapy, some patients will get what's called radiation proctitis, or rectal pain. That's a delayed reaction that's kind of a vascilitis from the radiation therapy. It can cause pain, sometimes bleeding, and can be, in rare cases, quite disabling. Fortunately, that's not a common occurrence, but it does happen. We have seen that most often in combination of external beam radiation therapy plus brachytherapy. Those are the patients that are more likely to have a serious complication from the therapy.

One of the key treatments for prostate cancer is radiation, an energy source. It changes the cellular structure of the tumors to kill them, but the surrounding tissue also receives some of the effect. The radiation therapy that's given nowadays is more precise than it was twenty years ago. We're seeing a lot fewer side effects than we used to see.

Somewhere along the line of six months to a year after a patient finishes radiation, we might see his PSA go up a bit then go back down. We call this a PSA bounce. If a PSA goes up and stays up we will do a prostasint scan to look for recurrent disease.

In radiation therapy, we notice a lot of fatigue. It's a common occurrence. Many patients turn the corner at six months. To help, I encourage them to stay active. You can get out of condition very quickly at an advanced age, or any age for that matter. You'll never get back to where you were if you don't work at it.

There's also an element of depression that goes with it. There are medications to take for that, and probably a multi-vitamin will help. An exercise program that begins even before the therapy and continues through it is also important to recovery.

"Our research team has found that Rapamycin, a promising anti-cancer drug in its own right, dramatically impairs the generation of life-sustaining energy by late-stage prostate cancer cells.

"Therefore, we may soon be treating prostate cancer patients with Rapamycin and other drugs that disrupt the energy-producing machinery in cancer cells while they are undergoing radiotherapy. We are optimistic that co-treatment with agents like Rapamycin will increase the efficacy and decrease the side effects of radiation therapy in patients with prostate cancer."

— *Robert Abraham, Ph.D.*
Director, Cancer Research Center,
The Burnham Institute

Denis E. Waitley, Ph.D.—prostate cancer
Sixty-nine years old—Rancho Santa Fe, California
Author of best selling Psychology of Winning; *management consultant*

On a Sunday in 1994, the *San Diego Union* ran an ad promoting free PSA tests at Scripps Hospital. I said, "Why not do it, it's free." So I moseyed on over to Scripps and took the PSA. They did both the digital and the blood test. The digital said no problems, nice and smooth as silk. Yet the PSA came back at about 5.0. I watched it for a couple of months and it went up to 6.0, so I decided to begin my own investigative process.

I went to the Mayo Clinic, Stanford University, John's Hopkins, and really started getting into it. I had a biopsy at Mayo, and it came back positive. The urologist said, "You have a garden variety of prostate cancer. It's not too big right now, but we recommend instant surgery."

At that particular point, Johns Hopkins was doing several a day. They were surgeons, they were good, and they said, "We try to spare the nerves." I tried to go a little deeper into it, so I went to Stanford University and had a biopsy. Sure enough, my prostate was pretty big and there was a small pea-size tumor.

I asked each of these great people who had written papers and were leading authorities in the field, "If I was your son, what would you recommend?" They said that was an unfair question because you need to make your own decisions about your body and your life with qualified professional input. I said, "I understand that, and I understand malpractice. You don't want to get too personally involved with me and tell me exactly what you would do if you were me." So they just gave me my options.

My Gleason number was low, which meant it was not growing and multiplying really rapidly, at least in my case. Some doctors recommended radical prostatectomy, which Johns Hopkins was doing, that involved more sparing of the nerves. Mayo said they could do it with more sparing of the nerve endings, but none of them could tell me whether I would be incontinent or impotent.

At that particular time, I had just signed a one million dollar contract to speak almost every day in 1995. I could plan the tour starting in the south and going up to the north. It would begin in February and end in November. It was a contract I had signed in conjunction with promoting my new book.

I distinctly remember the Mayo urologist saying, "Don't barter your life for money." I, of course, said, "I'm not going to do that, but I've signed a contract and I feel great." I'm an assertive guy; I want to make the right decision. He said, "Just be careful, you're looking at the money." I said, "You know, I am probably going to go on tour." He said, "You should wait a year, because I really can't say what will happen in that twelve-month period of time."

A cover article in *Fortune* had just been published on Andrew Grove, the chairman and founder of Intel, and it was a whole story about what he did when he was diagnosed with cancer. I read the article with a certain amount of interest and passion because he went to the same urologist and leaders in the field as I had. He mentioned in the article about meeting with the doctors, what they told him he should do, and what a friend told him to do and what someone else recommended, and it basically came down to his decision. He decided to do something different. He chose the brachytherapy. It was a relatively new procedure using computer guided hollow straws that are placed directly around the tumor in the prostate. Then, extremely high doses of iridium are inserted into those straws.

After I read the article, I started picturing myself being on the road, speaking everyday, and having to deal with the urgency to urinate, along with being impotent. I visualized having to say, "I think there is somebody waving their hands in the back of the auditorium with an urgent phone call for me." Then I'd run off the stage to the men's room and run back. I'm not sure whether or not it was the right decision, but I elected to have brachytherapy, the same procedure that Andrew Grove chose. I reasoned that since he was a billionaire and a scientist, and since he had done a lot of heavy research, it was a wise choice.

I went to the Swedish Hospital in Seattle, where they inserted the hollow straws around the tumor in the prostate. I got to see it on an MRI, which was really funny because as I looked though the machine to see the doctors manipulating the straws, my penis was visible right against one doctor's forehead. So I asked, "Is this what dick-head means?" The doctor shot back, "That really isn't funny, and we don't need that kind of comment now." He had no sense of humor.

They insert this little platform with the straws in it, and the next day they take you down to what looks like a milking machine where they give you a high dose of iridium. They only go in for a fraction of a second, and then they zap it. I had two of those sessions. There's no fatigue whatsoever after the high dose; there is nothing you feel from that except the discomfort when they remove the straws.

The toughest part is removing those hollow straws because they are inserted directly in the prostate, and there are a number of them. It is what I would imagine giving birth to a large child and passing a kidney stone at the same time would be like. They told me that they were going to tug on this thing and that it would feel like my insides were coming out, and it did.

I went back to Scripps Hospital and had the thirty-day external beam radiation, which I'm sure cooked most of my glands and organs around the prostate. I didn't have any side effects, other than the normal ones.

I'm now in my eighth year. My PSA was 0 for about five years and it's now 0.1. I don't know what the long-term outcome is going to be, but I'm very careful. I watch my diet, and I get my PSA checked every four months.

One interesting thing to come out of this is that I noticed that men never want anyone to know they have any weakness or sickness that puts them at a disadvantage in their competition with other males. So men, generally speaking, hesitate to reveal their feelings and emotions. We don't want to show any vulnerability to our peers. Remember, big boys don't cry. But this event did give me a wake-up call and made me realize I'm mortal.

All through my life, when I haven't felt good, I've crawled off by myself. I didn't want anyone attending to me. I didn't want anyone to say anything or feel sorry for me. I certainly didn't want anyone caring for me. If you live this way, you end up being an arrogant, stoic warrior. That is, until somebody tells you, "Hey buddy, you have a garden variety of prostate cancer."

"One thing about prostate cancer is you're not alone. You have your own support group all around you: doctors, family and friends. However, you have to take the first step and open up to them."

— *Charlie Jones—prostate cancer,*
co-author

Steve Smith—prostate cancer
Sixty-one years old—Seal Beach, California
Executive with Lehman Brothers

I have a problem with prostate cancer. After I had a prostatectomy, which was the modality of choice during my prognoses/diagnosis, they didn't get it all. The PSA should have been post-prostatectomy 0.00, but instead it was 1.8. The surgeon, however, felt that he had gotten it all. There was no evidence of the cancer having broken the capsule, and the pathology of the lymph nodes and the surrounding tissues that he removed showed absolutely no evidence of cancer. He was very, very optimistic two days or so after the surgery, especially since I'm in fairly good health and have the bloodline of Mr. Stan Smith, the Wimbledon and U.S. Open tennis champion. (I'm his older brother.)

However, as soon as the doctors saw that I was not cured, which, of course, is the goal of surgery, they took six cores—each one was fairly saturated with the disease. Immediately after that result, they put me on hormonal therapy for a year to cut the testosterone production, which is the fuel that feeds the disease.

Then in March of 2002, my PSA got to almost 1.0 and I went back on Lupron and Casodex. Casodex is a pill, an expensive little bugger. My PSA went down from almost 1.0 to 0.2, which was encouraging. But by August, it was up again. The last PSA I took was 0.8.

Knowing that my PSA had gone up, my oncologist suggested that I not continue with Casodex, which primarily affects the production of testosterone in my adrenal glands, to see if my PSA will go down. At the end of the month, I'll have another PSA taken and if it has gone down from 0.8, that's a good sign. But if it's at that level or larger, then they're going to test me again at the end of October. If it stays up, I'll be a candidate for some sort of an experimental drug, which is not available to people who are otherwise getting along fine with hormonal therapy.

My original story began, maybe five years ago, when I had a bladder infection and it was really painful to pee. I went to my doctor—I've never been sick in my life—and he gave me little pills to correct the infection. Then he said, "Have you ever had a PSA taken?" I said, "No, but I've flown PSA (Pacific Southwest Airlines)."

I just wasn't aware. The PSA was relatively new in the history of medicine. It came out in the 1980s. He said, "You shouldn't have your PSA taken after you've taken medication, so later on you should see an oncologist." I did, and my PSA was 3.84, which is near the 4.0 threshold. He said, "You should come back and have it tested and see where you are." I didn't know anything about the 4.0 or the disease, so I didn't go back.

Then about three years ago, I said, "Gee, I haven't had that PSA taken. Maybe I better go get a physical and that PSA thing." So I went back to the same doctor, and my PSA came out 12.6. That was within three years. He told me he needed to take a biopsy. Afterward he called and said, "When can you come in? I need to talk with you about your biopsy. Bring your wife." Not a good sign. He gave both of us the story and gave me a shot of Lupron on the spot. Then we talked about modalities. Of course, he's a surgeon. If you want bread, go to a baker, right?

I researched prostate cancer from coast to coast, including who were the top doctors in the country, and decided on surgery as my best choice. So about three months later, I went under the knife. In the meantime, I was on Lupron and Casodex, and my PSA was dropping. It went from 12.6 down to about 5.0.

I had the surgery and recovered. I could've gotten out the day after the operation. I felt pretty good, a little uncomfortable with the catheter, but I had the surgery on a Monday morning and on Friday I was in an electronics store buying some stuff for my computer. I just couldn't sit still.

My sex life has gone from fairly active to zero. They took out the nerves, so I have a little limp weenie. Emotionally, though, I'm fine. I think about it a lot. I can see the wall. I work out a couple times a week, I play tennis with my son and grandson. I'm not a great player, never was. However, the last time I played Stan I beat him. (editorial note: Steve was eighteen years old, Stan was thirteen.)

From an emotional point of view, I know that I have a real serious situation, but I'm not that special. I have a philosophy that we're all going to die, it's just a matter of when. All I can do is what I can do. When I got the prognosis, I went on a strict vegetarian diet. I eliminated, as much as possible, animal products from my diet. I'm a slacker and I'll have fish and maybe chicken once in a while. My wife isn't as crazy as I am. She's a little bit of a cynic.

I bought a juicer; the Norlock juicer, which is a $2,000 machine. I juice vegetables and pineapples and stuff like that. I try to eat well, and I try to keep my stress level down. Actually, part of the therapy is talking about it. It's also giving of yourself to other people. So I've become an evangelist, of sorts, on lifestyle. My wife was an agnostic before all this happened, but now she can quote Bible verses, although she's quick to mention that it's not necessarily the Christian religion that would work for everyone. It's just a matter of getting into your spiritual self. A lot of it is in the mental area.

I don't think about dying. I don't let myself think about it. I listen to my body. I just wonder whether this ache and that pain is the beginning of some kind of a bone disease, if cancer has invaded my bones. How I feel today: Is this the best that I'm ever going to be for the rest of my life? I think about that once in a while, but then again, I could be hit by a truck.

"In some ways, having prostate cancer was a very, very formative experience, meaning that it made me ask questions—that made it possible to get through September 11th better—about life and death, mortality, the fact that you have to live every day with the possibility you're going to die, whether you have cancer or you don't. Somebody who has cancer and has to treat it and overcome it has just been more dramatically confronted with that possibility."

— *Rudy Giuliani—prostate cancer,*
former mayor of New York City

Bill Potts—Prostate cancer
Sixty-seven years old—Huntington, New York
President, The Creative Consortium, Ltd.

They discovered my prostate cancer in 1998, and I went through the whole process that you go through. The hardest part was trusting that you were given a straight story about the options you had. As a matter of fact, I just got off the phone with my friend Bill Meredith, president of Cinesound, who has prostate cancer, and he said the same thing. The hardest part was finding the medical advice he could really trust and have faith in.

I wound up selecting the road with no surgery, which meant the combination of radiation, hormone therapy and radioactive implants, which turned out to be 100 percent successful. I never, ever had any discomfort. However, I did have some reaction from the hormone therapy. You actually go into menopause and start having hot flashes in the middle of the night, and you get a little emotional about things. You have more intuition, and your sex life goes to hell in a hand basket. You stop growing hair and you get boobs.

The other thing I had to address was whether to tell people or to keep it a big secret. I think cancer patients who right away say, "Okay, I've got it and it's under control," or "It's a problem, but I'm dealing with it," seem to have much more successful outcomes than those who pretend there is nothing going on.

I was amazed by the number of people who came out of my past and wanted to help. For some obscure reason, I got tons of cookbooks. Being a bachelor, my idea of weekly shopping is a half case of Spam and a half case of red wine. Friends were introducing me to green things, and lots of tomatoes. In fact, I wound up changing my diet.

After my treatment, I made a big effort to keep myself very busy, forcing myself not to dwell on my cancer. I knew there wasn't anything I could do about it. Every time my next PSA rolled around, three months, six months, nine months, and then a year, the number just kept getting lower and lower. I made an effort to put it out of my mind, forget about it and get on with life and accept the fact that you probably don't ever get over cancer. You just put it in remission. Besides, they have a hell of a track record; they pretty much guarantee ten years with the radiation treatment.

I've had a number of friends who have been diagnosed with cancer and just collapsed the minute they heard the "C" word. My mom had cancer and the minute she heard the word, that was it, it was a death sentence. No matter what anybody told her. She had a doctor who she really trusted. He was her oldest friend and he said, "Once we identify it, we'll go after it and get rid of it." She would not believe that. There was no way in the universe she would buy that assumption. I think that may be true with older people because cancer was a death sentence not that many years ago.

People talk more about cancer now. It needs to be talked about it, and to be out in the open. I have heard conversations at parties, "Oh, he's in terrible trouble, he's got cancer." When I asked, "Of what?" They'd answer, "Well, you know, he hasn't told us." That person is collapsing inside himself like a big hole in a galaxy that is far, far away.

I think success comes down to just plain attitude. People who go out and get the best advice they can get from people they trust and then attack it, have the best chance to win. I don't see that it's any different than a broken arm or a case of the hives. You have to approach them all the same way. It's just that such an aura surrounds the word cancer that people whisper about it as the "Big C."

I've tried everything I can think of to forget about it and get on with my life. I made a conscious effort to do that, even to the degree that while I was in the doctor's office after the last check-up and he said, "Well now, I need to see you in a year, have you brought your calendar with you?" I said, "No, and I don't want to set a date. Send me a note or call me up when the time rolls around." I didn't want to look at my desk calendar and see my PSA test coming up. I used a quote from Atilio Luigi Ferdenzi, Jr. (The "Ashland Avalanche" scatback from Boston College): "Shove all the lions and tigers back in their cages." It worked. So far, I've been very happy. I even made a point of dealing with it in my Christmas letter.

Remember, with prostate cancer there is that old bugaboo about you don't want to talk about your genital parts in public. I think ladies run into the same problem when they don't want to talk about their breast cancer or cancer of what one ninety-year-old lady friend of mine refers to as her "gentleman's entrance."

I think a sense of humor has everything to do with it. It does have a funny side, which is the way people react to you and how you react yourself. You need to keep an eye peeled for the absurdity of it all because it does take up a disproportionate amount of your living time if you think about it. If you let people know that it hasn't beaten you down, it will in fact, turn out that it *hasn't* beaten you down. I wouldn't want to do it again, but it turned out to be a non-event in my life.

However, because I had the radioactive seed implant, I do get reminded that I'm a walking nuclear waste dump. When I get on and off of airplanes, my crotch sets off the alarm. Then I have to produce documentation, and if I say loudly, "I have seeds in my groin," they blush and stammer. They think it's a bomb and they start looking in my ear for a fuse, then they take me back to another room. To survive, all you have to do is have fun with it.

"From my research, I have determined that red wine is a curative for the loss of your sex drive from treatment for prostate cancer. In honor of medical science, I have tried to drink my share. I believe merlot is most effective."

> — *Prostate cancer survivor,*
> *name was smeared by a dark maroon,*
> *sticky substance*

Len Dawson—prostate cancer
Sixty-seven years old—Kansas City, Missouri
Kansas City Chiefs quarterback, Pro Football Hall of Fame,
Super Bowl IV MVP

Linda Dawson
Len's wife

I was reading the paper and saw this ad for a free PSA screening. For whatever reason, because I never do anything like that, I called and made an appointment for Len. This was during the football season. When he came home Thursday night from New York City after taping "Inside The NFL" for HBO, I said, "Honey, I got an appointment for you at 9:15 tomorrow morning to go for your PSA screening." He said, "What are you talking about?" I answered, "It's a prostate cancer screening, just a couple blocks away, and I set it up for you." In typical fashion, he responded, "I don't have any time." I said, "Look, if you're not going, you have to call and cancel it yourself because I'm not going to do it for you." I honestly don't know why I did it. I never do that with Len.

Len Dawson

I got lucky. I came home from out of town and Linda said, "I want you to read this article about Senator Bob Dole, who found out he had prostate cancer through his PSA test." This was in 1991, when the PSA test was relatively new. I read the story about how Senator Dole's PSA test was elevated and that led to the discovery that he had cancerous tumors. He had the radical surgery. I said, "What's that got to do with me?" Linda replied, "Did you read the symptoms?" I said, "Yeah, but I don't have any of the symptoms."

On the same page was an advertisement promoting free PSA tests and stating that anybody over fifty who hadn't had this screening should get it done. It's an indicator to determine if there could be a problem with prostate cancer. Linda had made an appointment for me, but I told her I was too busy and felt fine. Needless to say, I went.

I took the PSA and they were going to get the results back to me in a week or two. I was about to leave when a nurse said, "If you'll step in the office, the doctor will complete the examination," which meant a rectal examination. He found something and thought I should have an ultrasonic image and a biopsy. They discovered I had a tumor that was malignant, but not large, and they thought they had found it in the early stages.

My first reaction was shock, and my next reaction, because it had been implanted in my brain since childhood, was that this was it. How long was I going to be around? Fear is another thought that crossed my mind. Fear of the unknown.

Because I didn't know the doctor in Kansas City, I wanted a second opinion. I went to Memorial Sloan-Kettering in New York City, which has the reputation as the finest cancer hospital in the world, and they concurred that I had prostate cancer.

I had three options. One, that I didn't do anything, which didn't make much sense to me. Two was radiation, and three was surgery. They have developed a new nerve-saving technique in surgery, and you don't have that choice if you have radiation; so I opted for surgery.

One of the reasons I chose this option was because my oldest brother Ron died of prostate cancer a few years ago, and his only choice was radiation. He was one of those guys who didn't talk much. He was a paratrooper in the Normandy invasion, got hit with shrapnel, was captured, and the next day the Americans took over and he was still alive, so he came back. He never talked about his experiences over there, and he never talked about his prostate cancer, but he should have. I was fortunate. They got it early. I got lucky, but that's what I expect. After all, I am the seventh son of a seventh son.

Former Buffalo Bills coach Marv Levy called me when he found out he had prostate cancer. He knew I had gone through it. I told him to get a second opinion, just to make sure that somebody else concurs with the doctor who examined you.

Marv got a second opinion and he, too, opted for surgery. I asked him, "Why surgery?" Marv was in his seventies and some men, when they get to a certain age, decide not to do anything because prostate cancer is slow growing. But Marv, like me, said, "I want it out of my body."

What I found out about cancer is that I can handle it. I played football for all those years and my body knows that I can handle it, but I also found out cancer affects everybody who cares about you. My wife was apprehensive when she made that appointment. She thought she had done something wrong. I told her, "Honey, you saved my life."

Linda Dawson
Len's wife

Why in the world would I ever, out of the blue, make an appointment for some exam for Len? I still don't know what prompted me to do it. It was just so strange, because Len would not have done it on his own. It was just such a weird thing. He had a radical prostatectomy and after that, he has felt just fine. That was in 1991.

Name withheld by request—prostate cancer
Mid-sixties—Chicago, Illinois
Retired surgeon

If I was seventy-five years old and had the same diagnosis, I wouldn't have done anything. I'd probably have them shoot me with a couple of hormone shots to block out Testosterone effects. At that age, more than likely, you'll die of another cause. Ninety-eight to 99 percent of men by age ninety will have had prostate cancer. That's how Mother Nature reacts with those cells. But the treatment question is, what age and what kind of tumor? Right now, no one has that answer. The only thing is, you're not going to treat someone seventy or over the same way as if they're fifty-five or sixty.

I had the diagnosis but didn't have surgery for a couple of months. I wanted to collect my blood. As a doctor, I knew, from having done it for other patients for all those years, that I wanted to get two units regardless of what they told me. I'm glad I did because I needed them. I knew that was going to take a six-week period, so I had essentially two months before surgery.

Anyway you look at it, they had to do all the exams and CT scans. But I had a bone scan, and that was negative, so it relieved my anxiety because I then knew the cancer hadn't moved into my bones. That's just one good sign. Then subsequently, I had the CT scans, and those were also negative.

There's an advantage to being a doctor when one has five negative biopsies and one positive, because you think, My God, at least it's not throughout the prostate gland. It seemed to be confined because they could only find one little area out of six biopsies. But in your own mind's eye view, as a doctor, you know too damned much about what happens with metastatic disease, and that all you really need is one little cell to slip out of there.

You're really uptight until you have your bone scan. It makes a big difference when the bone scan is negative. Then you can relax a little bit and figure, well, at least it's not in my bones. But until you get your CT scan and realize it's not outside the confines of prostate, it's a staging type thing. You are uptight until each particular diagnostic test is done.

I was lucky because all my nodes were negative. My cancer was contained to the capsule, so I figured I'd just have to wait and see. There's uncertainty, to say the least, for the first year after surgery. The question is what your PSA is going to be. When the whole tumor is taken out and the prostate is taken out, you're supposed to have a negative PSA. Mine has been negative for two years. Yet, the questions remain. Were there some cells that weren't contained? Did some escape the capsule? And even though my seminal vesicles were negative and my nodes were negative, who knows what's out there. I am always thinking about such things.

The thing I had to struggle with most postoperatively was having a catheter in me for three weeks. I had spasms in my urethra that were unbelievable. I had to stand there in excruciating pain, thirty times a day. I would just go into spasm. I couldn't do anything about it. But fortunately, they wouldn't last too long. I'd count to thirty, and by that time they were usually gone.

I was able to function on five to six hours of sleep. That was my modus operandi. But two months after surgery, I still couldn't get enough sleep. It really took me four months to feel pretty decent. My main problem was my urine control. I didn't have good urine control until about a year after the surgery. I wore diapers for six months.

I'll never forget when I first started playing golf, I'd wear dark clothes. Everything I wore was dark, even my shorts. There wasn't a tree I didn't love, particularly ones with big trunks I could hide behind.

I had the nerve-sparing surgery, which is rather a recent approach. It was successful and therefore I have had very little loss in my erectile capacity. It's not what it once was, but I'm doing just fine.

"The day the catheter was taken out was one of the happiest days of my life."

— *David Cooper—prostate cancer,*
retired columnist

"When you're told you have cancer, you've got to deal with it yourself and you've got to figure out how to be alone with yourself and come to terms with it; come to terms with the fact that it's a deadly disease."

— *Rudy Giuliani—prostate cancer,*
former mayor of New York City

Bennie Bickers—prostate cancer
Sixty years old—Dallas, Texas
Retired from the securities business

When the PSA test first came out, I told my doctor that I wanted it to be included in my blood work. After seeing him a year later, he called and said "This is probably nothing, but your PSA has gone up a full point in one year and you need to see a specialist." My dad died of cancer so I said, "I'll do that right away."

I went to the doctor and they took a biopsy and when it came back they said, "Yes, it is cancer." They told me that more than likely it was completely contained inside the prostate. Then the doctor gave me what I thought was one of the most idiotic set of options I've ever heard. (Of course, I knew nothing about cancer.) He said I could have my prostate completely removed or I could have radiation or I could wait and see.

I said, "Wait and see what? Wait and see if it spreads?" He replied, "Well, yes." But I said, "That's not an option. Explain the other two." He told me, "Radiation is not as invasive as surgery, but if the cancer returns, that's all we can do for you. But if we do surgery and the prostate is taken out and the cancer returns, we can still radiate." I said, "There's really only one option, unless you want to live with cancer inside of you, and I don't know anybody in their right mind who would opt for that."

He operated the following Thursday and I checked out of the hospital at noon on Saturday. I didn't have much trouble at all with incontinence and as far as being impotent, that was a fact for a while. That was even before Viagra, but now they have three or four different other things so that if you still have the desire, you can still have sex.

I was careful to get a physical every year for five years, but I haven't seen a doctor in a year and a half now. However, if there is any sign of my PSA going up, I'll change that in a hurry. I'll hot-foot-it to get some tests run. But so far so good.

The worst thing that happened to me during all of this was when my catheter bag came apart at a cocktail party. Thank God, I was with close friends. They all started looking at my leg. I glanced down and the catheter had separated from the bag and all my pee was everywhere. I had not even realized it, and I had light colored sweats on. The hostess casually said, "Let me get my son-in-law to find you another pair of sweats."

Mostly now, I get calls from people who have been diagnosed with cancer. I'll spend all day on the phone with them or go meet them. I don't try to sugarcoat it but try to tell them how easy a time it can be; it's only as hard as you make it.

I went to get a haircut this morning, and because I got laid off this past November from the securities business, my barber asked me, "Are you still in the ranks of the unemployed?" I said, "I sure am." He said, "Are you starting to worry about it?" And I said, "You know, Tom, sometimes when I'm leaving the golf course, I'll recall having to be in the office." However, it really does bother me not having that big paycheck at the end of every month, but I've finally gotten old enough not to worry about things I can't control. A computer tape does what I used to do. I'm not ever going to get that back so why worry about it?

Gene Burroughs—prostate cancer
Seventy years old—San Diego, California
Investment advisor

I'd like to mention something that you're never told, but doctors will admit happens if you have prostate surgery. When they take this thing like a walnut out, which shortens your tubing, it pulls up your genitals and your testicles. The result, in effect, is that while most men all their life wish they had a penis that was one inch longer, after prostate surgery, you end up with one that's an inch shorter.

I told my doctor, "I feel like you took something away from me," just teasing. I asked, "Have there been any studies?" He said, "There are no studies on this. Nobody talks about it, but I know that it happens." There are certain types of surgery men will have to lengthen their penis. The way they do that is they go up and cut off a little bit of the infrastructure that holds it inside, and actually bring it outside.

The reverse is happening here. They've gone inside and cut out part of your infrastructure. It brings you back up inside. So, as a man, you end up with less of a penis than you had before, which psychologically affects you a little bit. Those are the kinds of things, obviously, a mature person lives with. You're really grateful for the solutions they have, but they don't always tell you about these things.

This is kind of unbelievable, but within ten days after surgery, I could experience an erection. Let me tell you what happens. Doctors pride themselves on what they call nerve-sparing surgery. There are two sets of nerves, one has to do with your urine/bladder, and the other has to do with your sexual function. These nerves are about the size of hairs. So they're dealing with stuff that's very demanding. I was very fortunate in that the doctor preserved those hair-sized nerves, apparently related to my sexual function.

However, he was not able to preserve the nerves related to the incontinence (leaking urine). Did that affect me sexually? Yes. What happens is, as my wife and I are preparing to have a relationship, we begin to think sexually. The message comes down to my pelvic area: relax, enjoy yourself. When it gets that message of relaxation, the urine begins to flow and, obviously that affects your sexual relationship because you want to take a clean body to your wife. You don't want to take one that has urine all over it. So it has affected us. At our age and our maturity, we live with it. There are other satisfactions. You kind of work your way around it. But it does affect you; there's no question about that.

Bill Espy—prostate cancer
Seventy-six years of age—Prattville, Alabama
Retired Lt. Colonel, U.S.A.F., OSI

I cope with my cancer one day at a time. The operation was tough. It's a pretty serious operation. You wouldn't think so, but it is. This was in 1996. When they took out my prostate, the margins were not clear, which indicates that the cancer was not contained. So, we waited until I got over the operation to begin radiation. After about three months, we began the thirty-six treatments of radiation. I took the attitude that I wasn't going to let it get me down.

I had an awful lot of support. My oldest son came for a week, then my next son came for a week, and then my next. They really took care of me as far as support is concerned.

After the radiation, I didn't have any energy. I still don't have any. I play golf, but instead of playing eighteen holes, I'll play nine. I can get by with that. But playing eighteen just completely wears me out.

I don't have any real bad days; mine are all just about the same. I do what I'm going to do in the morning. When we play golf, we play at about seven o'clock in the morning. For one thing, in this part of the country, it's a little cooler then. In the afternoon, I just don't do anything but read or watch television.

We do travel, particularly to see the kids. We stay home about three months and then travel a month. We've got a bunch of grandkids, and we go out there and take care of them for a couple of weeks. You'd be surprised what you can do with the grandkids. You just don't have time to think about what is bothering you. On top of that, I got shingles about six months ago. My doctor caught them right at the very beginning, and I'll be damned if I still don't have the post-neuralgia part. He says I'll probably have it for about eighteen months.

We're getting ready to go see our oldest son, who is in Seattle now, and hell, we're just going to do it. I'm going to do everything I can while I can still do it. I think you'll find as time goes on, you'll gain some of your strength back. Then you won't have those bad days and good days. As I said, mine are pretty much all the same.

"I have talked with some patients who had chemo rather than radiation. They preferred chemo because of the side effects. They felt more like they were fighting cancer."

— *Dr. David Hodgens,*
Medical Director of Radiation
Oncology, Scripps Memorial Hospital

Clint Murchison III—prostate cancer
Fifty-five years old—Dallas, Texas
Businessman

After going through a blood test and then a biopsy, I had a radical prosta-tectomy in August of 1998. The worst part was the catheter. I had that for two weeks. As I describe it, it's like having a clothespin attached to your pecker, and you're carrying it around. That was very unpleasant. I was extremely weak for the first week or ten days. Then after that, I got better and better. I played golf less than forty days after the operation. The doc-tor didn't say, "Don't do it." But then, I didn't ask.

I had almost no after-effects. None. I was very lucky. Supposedly, most people have incontinence. I experienced a very minor amount. I never had to wear a diaper. As for sexual function, it had no effect on me. As I said, I've been extremely fortunate.

I didn't know that much about prostate cancer and I kept thinking about the odds that they told me when I got my blood test. "Your chances of having prostate cancer are such and such percent." Then when they did the biopsy, they told me that my chances of having operable prostate can-cer are such and such percent. I kept looking at those numbers, and every time, I fell in the positive range.

It just kept coming and I really didn't know what to think. But I figured I've got to go through this process. I don't want to, but what's the alterna-tive? So I just did it. It turned out okay. There wasn't any great fear or regret, or whatever else goes along with finding out that you have cancer. It was just one of those things: a challenge in life that you have to face. My attitude is that we're all going to go someday; some of us are just going to go sooner than others.

Herbert York, Ph.D.—prostate cancer and acute leukemia
Eighty-and-a-half years old—La Jolla, California
(When I mention this people say, "Only children count their ages five, five-and-a-half, six, six-and-a-half." I reply, "When you get to be eighty you'll do it again.")
Nuclear physicist, presidential advisor, Enrico Fermi Award recipient

I'm in a thirteen-year remission from prostate cancer and a two-year remission from acute leukemia. After a lot of soul searching, I had radiation for my prostate cancer. It came back in just over three years. I then went on hormone therapy, and that has worked beautifully for eight years.

The principle effect of the radiation was to really knock down my energy level quite severely. I didn't do anything to combat this except to behave in a normal way, and eventually my energy returned.

At this point, I suddenly realized that life has other lessons. So my wife and I flew to Hong Kong, first class, and we stayed in the Mandarin Hotel. We decided that elegance was deserved under those circumstances.

The chemo for leukemia really knocks you out much more severely than radiation. I lost all my hair, but it came back delightfully, a little bit stiffer, but the same color and it covers the same part of my head. Now I encourage all women to run their fingers through it. I've been doing that since I was eighty-and-a-half years old.

Dave Cox—prostate cancer
Sixty-four years old—Sacramento, California
Minority Republican Leader of the California Assembly

I was diagnosed with prostate cancer in 1997. I had twenty-five days of radiation and then had the seed implant. I've had some friends who had prostate cancer and then ten years later it came back.

The interesting thing about prostate cancer is that to date there is no cure. If the cancer gets out of the prostate gland, the chances of it returning and metastasizing in some other organ is a real possibility. It may take five, ten, or fifteen years before this happens. If it has escaped, it causes all kinds of problems.

But, if the cancer is contained in the prostate gland and hasn't spread beyond it, that's the best news of all. By the way, the number of men with prostate cancer in California tracks almost evenly with women who have breast cancer. The brotherhood and sisterhood is large, and getting larger.

Chris Foster, M.D.—prostate cancer
Seventy years old—San Diego, California
Retired physician (ear, nose, and throat specialist)

I had proton radiation for prostate cancer and had my most inconvenience from the frequency of my urination and from Pyridium, the medication for urine irritation. It turns the color of your urine to a bright reddish-orange, and it stains everything it touches. We were constantly cleaning up. It's an old medicine; they were using it when I started medical school back in 1953.

I find that the best way of handling my cancer is keeping myself distracted—reading a book, going to a movie, watching television. I'm also playing tennis again.

"The tennis may have had something to do with my recovery. I was in great shape. I had a positive attitude when I went to my radiation at 7:45 in the morning. After that I went directly to the Del to teach. I didn't miss one day of work."

> — *Ben Press—prostate cancer,*
> *tennis pro at the Hotel Del Coronado in*
> *California for twenty-eight years*

Name withheld by request—prostate cancer
Akron, Ohio
Retired newspaperman

My doctor said from the start that there could be erection problems. "If there's a problem, we'll fix it," he said. Several weeks after the surgery, he gave me Viagra to try. Well, the Viagra has not worked yet, so I am, per my doctor's instructions, doing injection therapy.

If anyone had ever suggested that I would inject my dingus with a syringe about halfway down, I would have said they were nuts. However, it works like a charm, so well, in fact, that I have had a three-hour stiffy each time I have done it, which is about once a week. Some scheduling is essential, as you cannot comfortably smuggle one of those hard-ons into a dinner party.

"Viagra is like an amusement park. A forty-five-minute wait for a three-minute ride."

> — *Bennie Bickers—prostate cancer,*
> *retired securities analyst*

"Men who have trouble with erections after surgery or radiation therapy for prostate cancer can achieve a normal orgasm. This problem, called erectile dysfunction (ED), can always be treated."

> — *Dr. Patrick Walsh,*
> *Professor of Urology, The Johns*
> *Hopkins Medical Institutions*

Arnold Palmer—prostate cancer
Seventy-three years old—Latrobe, Pennsylvania, and Bay Hill, Florida
Legendary professional golfer

I have really been fortunate. Right after I was diagnosed with prostate cancer, I flew my plane to the Mayo Clinic in Rochester, Minnesota. They operated on Wednesday and on Friday, I flew home to Florida. I didn't have any problems and six weeks later, I started playing golf again.

As a cautionary procedure, I later had radiation, just to be sure that everything was covered. I had a slight energy loss but I played golf every day while I was taking radiation.

When anyone asks me about what I recommend, I always tell them to first make a decision on how they want to be treated, and then get it done. Don't fool around.

"It's somewhat shocking when you find out you have prostate cancer. It happens to other people; you just never think it's going to happen to you. I had surgery and now, knock on wood, it's as good as it can get. Prostate cancer comes with age. The key is early detection and I'd like to be an advocate for that. When a man gets to be fifty, he needs to have his PSA checked twice a year."

— *Raymond Floyd—prostate cancer,*
four-time PGA Tour major champion

"African Americans have the highest rates of prostate cancer in the world and are 50 percent more likely to develop it than men of other racial and ethnic groups. As a prostate cancer survivor, I urge men to take action. Don't take your health for granted. Take a more proactive role in your life. It's time to knock this disease out of the park. Early detection saves lives. It saved mine."

— *Dusty Baker—prostate cancer,*
manager of the Chicago Cubs

"I knew when I was ready to go back to work after my treatment for prostate cancer. That time came when I could stay awake after nine o'clock at night. That's when I knew I wouldn't fall asleep in the dugout."

— *Joe Torre—prostate cancer,*
manager of the New York Yankees

chapter six
Attitude-Attitude-Attitude

"Attitude" is the answer, the only answer. So simple, yet so difficult to accomplish. Some cancer survivors are born with the right attitude. It's their outlook on life. If it's not yours, then you better get with it because you'll need it to survive. "Attitude" is the most important word in this book.

———————————————

"Before cancer, I was always worrying about what I was going to be doing five or six years down the road. It's a terrible way to live. When I was sickest, I just decided I'm never going to waste another today thinking about tomorrow. This is it. Today is all I have."

— *Lance Armstrong—fourteen malignant tumors in his testicles, lungs and brain, four-time Tour de France champion*

John Mendelsohn, M.D.
Sixty-six years old—Houston, Texas
President of the University of Texas, M.D. Anderson Cancer Center

Part of fighting cancer is science, and part of it is attitude. Science is moving along great. We're able to do a lot more now than we ever could, and there are new things coming along.

But I don't think we know as much about how to help in strength and attitude as we should. A lot of that has to come from the individual. The doctor can be a catalyst and a guide and a helper and a friend. But it's an incredible challenge to someone who gets cancer. I really respect how they handle it.

"Maintain a positive attitude, and that will get you more mileage for your buck than any other treatment modification."

> — *Richard Hall, M.D., F.A.C.S.,*
> *Diplomate of the American Board of*
> *Urology*

"Every day that you're alive is one more day that they're moving towards a cure for cancer. My job is to be around long enough for them to find that cure, and I plan on doing that."

> — *Dave Cox—prostate cancer,*
> *Minority Republican Leader of the*
> *California Assembly*

Stephen M. Krant, M.D., F.A.C.S.

Fifty-nine years old—La Jolla, California
American Board of Plastic Surgery (reconstructive surgery)

My wife Lynn and I set up The SK Institute, a non-profit organization, to help cancer survivors and others. Breast Cancer Night began in April of 2002, with fourteen women who were my patients. Word-of-mouth took over and it has grown to thirty to thirty-five women a month. We give free services and treatment to make the patient feel better about herself. Survivors are able to share their experiences about what they're going through and what they've been through.

Participants have the choice of what they want. They can have a manicure, a pedicure, or a facial. We also offer body wraps, Dead Sea mud wraps, exfoliating salt scrubs, Vichy showers, or Swedish massages. The idea is to totally relax them. It's a positive setting where one is nurtured by her own peers and fellow survivors, and it's all free.

The women have developed a tremendous camaraderie. The letters we've received from them have been riveting in terms of how it's helped them and how it's made them feel better. We've had forty-year breast cancer survivors and we've had women who are currently going through radiation and chemotherapy.

Following this success, we wanted to expand our program, so our next event was Prostate Cancer Night. Because we just had a friend die of melanoma, we'll soon have Melanoma Cancer Night. We are also planning Ovarian Cancer Night.

Our spa director stood up at the International Spa and Fitness Association meeting with 4,500 people in the audience and said, "My name is Kelly Costa. I'm spa director at SK Sanctuary in La Jolla. Let me tell you what we do." In five minutes, she told the audience what we were doing, and then she said, "I challenge all the other spas in the country to do the same thing, not only for your clients, but for all those who are cancer patients."

We've had a lot of people asking us how to do it and how to get it started, and the *Today Show* has even visited us. There is a spa in Seattle that is thinking about doing it and another one in Santa Barbara. It's special. It's my most fun night of the month. Sharing with patients as they talk about their experiences is a perfect way to help cancer survivors feel better about themselves.

There was one woman in her late seventies whose daughter brought her to Breast Cancer Night. She was about 5'3" with beautiful blue eyes, a wrinkly face, and she was in a white robe after just having had a treatment. She came over, looked up at me, and said, "You know, Dr. Krant, this is one of the nicest nights in my life." I've worked with her daughter, a scrub nurse at Scripps Hospital, for twenty years. I went to the hospital the next day and found out that this woman has metastatic breast disease; the cancer is throughout her bones. But here she was telling me that this was one of the nicest nights of her life.

We have a friend who's had breast cancer for twelve years on and off, and she came and spoke at one of our evenings. She said, "You're not going to believe this, but breast cancer is the best thing that has ever happened to me. My family is more together, and I get more love and respect than ever. It's made me step back and think about what life's all about and the value of life." So it's all of those things. We did it because we wanted to give back, and it just turned around and gave so much more back to us.

"When I was touring in "Hello Dolly," I was diagnosed with uterine cancer. I went right on with the show, and on Saturdays I'd fly to New York City for cobalt and chemotherapy treatment. If you keep working, at the end of the show, you either feel better or you're cured."

— *Carol Channing—uterine cancer,
legendary Broadway star*

Anne Wallace, M.D., F.A.C.S.

Forty-one years old—La Jolla, California
Director of the Breast Care Unit, UCSD's Moores Cancer Center

The attitude of the breast cancer patient is extremely important. There is enough knowledge now about breast cancer that a woman doesn't think she is going to die the second she hears the diagnosis. Most breast cancer patients know tons of women who are walking around who have had it. A patient may be scared, but she's not thinking about dying.

Certainly, breast cancer is very life disruptive, and the ones who can shake that off and say, "Okay. I'm going to get through this and a year from now I'll return to my normal life," usually have a better recovery. Also, I've found that cancer patients who have complete trust in their health care provider and believe it is a complete team effort of which they are a part, do better.

A breast cancer survivor must realize that she is a different person afterward. She has to live with that different person, physically and emotionally. The woman who wants everything back to normal and can't get a grip on the fact that her life has changed is the one who really struggles.

I believe the energy that is created by a positive attitude is energy that can be applied to fighting any type of cancer. We don't quite understand the science behind it, but I think that someday we will.

Paul A. Marks, M.D.

Seventy-six years old—New York, New York
President Emeritus of Memorial Sloan-Kettering Cancer Center and
Member, Sloan-Kettering Institute for Cancer Research

The attitude of the cancer patient is very important in a number of ways. One of the problems with cancer is that the treatment can be very difficult. The patient who is motivated and optimistic about the long-range success is more likely to be someone you can treat effectively.

A "go for it" attitude is also crucial in terms of the patient's general well being. Cancer is frequently associated with loss of appetite, nausea, and lack of energy. Therefore, maintaining a correct dietary intake and some kind of exercise program is essential in terms of maintaining your ability to withstand cancer treatments, which can be very rigorous.

"Just getting out of the house is major therapy, even if you merely go stand in your driveway."

— *Dr. Gerald Wahman,*
senior urologist, Sparks Medical Plaza

Maryann Rosenthal, Ph.D.
Fifty-four years old—La Jolla, California
Licensed clinical and consulting psychologist

One of the first things I always stress with any caregiver of a cancer patient is their attitude. They have to put themselves first. Caregivers feel the person they're caring for is going through so much that they don't have a right as a caregiver to have any sort of selfish feelings, which is completely untrue.

They have to put themselves first, they need to take care of themselves. They need to have a life to try to reduce their stress. They need to have outlets. They have a lot of loneliness as caregivers. They give and give and give and if there is nothing left for themselves, it can bring on depression.

We all have our breaking point. Caregivers can learn coping skills. That's what I'm there for. They need that support. You know that they're supporting the patient, but who's supporting them? They need advice because when they're just caring, caring, caring for someone, it's like their decisions get clouded through a filter.

Sometimes I see there is some conflict and they don't even know it. I'm seeing this conflict as coming from the fact that they need a break from each other. What they're doing is transferring their problems on to the fact that they're tired and exhausted. Oftentimes, they need to either take time with each other or away from each other. Sometimes I give them direct advice: "Yes, you're in this together, but you still have to have a little peace."

Keith Eck—massive stroke, heart attack, squamous cell cancer, plane crash, car totaled

Forty-seven years old—North County, California
Former NFL offensive lineman, financial planning consultant

My heart attack at age thirty ended my NFL career, and my massive stroke eight years later almost ended my life. But my attitude is always to be 100 percent positive. Sure, I'm a realist and there's the possibility I can die; but to me, there's no benefit in dwelling on that or even spending much time thinking about it because you can't control it. I'd rather put positive thoughts in my mind and just be the survivor.

The one thing I learned during my stroke rehab was that the medical arena doesn't really understand all the influence of the power of the brain and how much impact the brain and positive thinking have on recovery. I saw so many doctors who wanted to give patients limits such as, "You'll only be able to move this much," or "Just do this." So, many people bought into those limits, and that's as far as they could go.

However, I had others in my stroke program, some little old ladies in their eighties to younger kids, who wouldn't buy into those limits. They just decided they were going to keep on going. They made greater improvements than they were ever expected to make, all because of their mental outlook.

For my squamous cell cancer, I had chemotherapy every Monday. I'd go into the doctor's office and they'd treat me for two or three hours, and then I'd go off and do my thing. My first chemo treatment lasted four-and-a-half hours and it was really brutal. I came home and just felt lethargic. But then on the second night I woke up and was sick all through the night. I was dry heaving; I was a mess.

I continued to work at my job the whole time during chemo, and actually I had one of my better years with my financial planning practice. Working helped keep my mind off how bad I felt.

On typical days, I'd go into work in the morning, and then leave about 2:00–2:30 P.M. I'd come home and collapse in bed. I would try to eat something, and I'd usually fall asleep around 8:00–8:30 P.M. I'd repeat it the next day. I think working also helped me.

I discovered that my second day after the chemo would be the day that I would feel the worst. Then as the week progressed, I would feel better and better and then, sure enough, as soon as I started to really feel good, it was Monday, and I'd have to return and get treated again. But I figured the worse I felt the better it was because that meant the cancer was getting beat up the most.

My radiation wasn't that big a deal at the start but by the end, it was very painful. They told me that head and neck radiation is the most intense radiation they do. Basically, it turns your mouth into one big sore. Towards the end, even ketchup tasted too spicy to swallow. I was existing on luke-warm chicken soup without the chicken, just the broth. It was really tough at the end.

I looked at it as, what choice did I have? To me, if something negative is going to happen, I'd rather be as positive as possible for the time that I'm here and enjoy life rather than walk around being negative. That probably comes from my sports training. I don't know any other way. I think, too, that I have a very special life.

I said earlier, the reason I feel this way is, I'm a survivor—massive stroke, heart attack, squamous cell cancer, and that single engine Cessna airplane that we crashed on take-off at a little airport in Kern County, California. There was also the time when I fell asleep at the wheel and rolled my van four times down a mountain road into oncoming traffic. So I figure I must still be here for a reason. My mission is to survive these things and be an influence.

I think the biggest thing that we can do for ourselves is feed the right thoughts into our mind. Everybody gets scared and wonders if they're going to be the one to die from cancer. But just like your body thrives on the right food, so does your mind. If you feed the right thoughts to your mind, you will convince yourself you're going to be a survivor. Somebody's going to do it. You know as well as I do that there are stories of people out there who are doing the things that doctors told them they could never do, or living longer than the doctor told them they were going to. There are stories everywhere. We see them all the time.

To me, the most important thing you can do is feed your mind the right food. A lot of people will find they are stronger than they ever thought they could be. Just put the right food in your mind and you'll convince yourself.

We all have times when we doubt. That's okay. Whenever it crossed my mind, What if I don't make it? or Will I see my kids again? I just said, "Okay. That's enough of that," and I put those thoughts out of my mind. And I told myself, "Now let's start feeding on the right thoughts again." That's the only way I know how to do it. It's worked for me, and I know it will work for you.

"More than anything, my heart attack set the tone for my attitude and all the recoveries I've had. I had made it as a free agent in the NFL with George Allen, of "Over The Hill Gang" fame, and then with the New York Giants. It was finally the right time, the right place. Then I had my heart attack. Mentally, it was about as demoralizing a thing you could go through, but I really think that set the tone for my life. I said, 'Screw it, I have my capabilities and I'll just go out and do something else.'"

— *Keith Eck*

"Courage is about the management of fear, not the absence of fear."

— *Rudy Giuliani—prostate cancer,*
former mayor of New York City

"I thought this would be a good time to have it done and get it behind me. It's treatable. Why not treat it now? In this game, you always have different challenges. A goal? Yeah, I have a goal: To be here every day."

— *Don Baylor—multiple myeloma (bone*
marrow cancer), on starting his
chemotherapy treatments after being
diagnosed, New York Mets bench coach

Ron Reina—stage four small cell lung and liver cancer
Sixty-six years old—Encinitas, California
Retired, special assistant to the sheriff

I had been wheezing in my breathing for a couple of weeks, and when I tried to clear my throat, I couldn't. I was coughing a lot, especially at night. Between the wheezing and coughing, I wasn't getting much sleep. I assumed that it was a chest cold or virus, so I took a lot of over-the-counter medicine, but that didn't help.

About a week later, I had my annual physical and commented to the doctor about what I had been experiencing for the past three weeks. He took x-rays in his office and concluded I had walking pneumonia. He said, "Your right lung is filled with puss and mucus, and that's what is putting pressure on your trachea, your wind pipe." He also told me that since their office x-ray machine was not the latest equipment, he wanted me to have a CT scan.

When I returned to his office for a follow-up, my wife was with me, and he sat us both down and said, "You have stage four cancer of the right lung and it has spread to your liver. The cancer has come out of the lung around your breast plate area and has wrapped itself partially around your wind pipe, which is why you're wheezing and why you feel shortness of breath."

He immediately sent me to an oncologist who agreed with the diagnosis, and the following day did a biopsy. Two days later they confirmed what kind of cancer I had. Initially, he thought he would attack it with radiation. However, when he saw it was small-cell and not non-cell, he said that radiation wouldn't work; I would have to have chemotherapy.

The next day, I began my chemotherapy. I had treatments on Tuesday, Thursday, and Monday. The doctor said the chemo would not only attack the cancer, it would also clear up my pneumonia symptoms. And it really has. I'm now able to sleep straight though the night. I don't have any wheezing at all. I can walk upstairs without a problem and I cough very very little.

I have chemo three times a week, once a month. They warned me about possible side effects, such as nausea, exhaustion, sweats, or shakes. When I had my first chemo treatment, which was about three hours in length, I had an IV hooked up to a vein in my wrist. My wife came with me the first day, and we took a box lunch and had a picnic. The next day, I felt a little bit of nausea, about nine or ten in the morning, which lasted a couple of hours. However, I got busy with other stuff and forgot all about it. That's the only side effect I have had. Apparently that's a good sign because the doctor was ecstatic when he heard that.

Right off the bat, I didn't take the attitude of "Why me?" Instead, I said, "Screw it; it's why me because it's my turn." I'm not going to go in the tank about it. I'm not going to go into a slump. If I cash in my chips in six months, six years, or sixteen years, so be it. I have no control over that. I smoked for thirty-five years; ironically I quit six years ago. And now I get lung cancer.

Bob Chandler, a good friend, had prostate cancer a couple of years ago. We had lunch and he told me the way he deals with cancer: "Because I play a lot of golf, to me, cancer is just like playing golf. You ended up with a bad lie, but you've still got to play the damn thing. If you hit a tee shot in the rough, you can't pick it up and throw it out on the fairway. You've still got to play it. You still have fifteen or sixteen holes to play. You don't quit after one or two holes."

I thought that was an excellent analogy. I loved it. So that's my attitude. My wife and I are still going to play golf and we're still going to travel. Screw it. I'm going to ride this horse as long as I can.

"You can find inspiration no matter what you're up against."

— *Diane Geppi-Aikens—terminal brain*
cancer, 40 years old, Loyola (Md.),
women's lacrosse coach

Tom Condren—multiple myeloma
Seventy-three years old—Fort Smith, Arkansas
Sales representative for furniture companies

My cancer is very rare. It's called multiple myeloma. The University of Arkansas Research Cancer Center in Little Rock is the finest treatment center in the world for this disease. Nationally known Dr. Bart Barlogie is head of the department, and he's the best in the business.

Dr. Barlogie is there because of Sam Walton. Sam had cancer and developed multiple myeloma at the end. He was going to M.D. Anderson in Houston for his treatments. I guess Sam got tired of flying down to Houston every so often, so he finally said to Dr. Barlogie, "What would it take for you and your staff to move to Little Rock, Arkansas?"

Dr. Barlogie said, "Well, Mr. Walton, we're very happy here in Houston. M.D. Anderson gives us just about everything we want." Sam said, "Dr. Barlogie, you don't understand. This is a blank check. What does it take for you to move to Little Rock?" And that's how he moved.

I was diagnosed in April of 2000. I didn't even know what myeloma was. It's a cancer of the blood and the bone. It's very serious, not curable, but treatable. The treatment that Little Rock uses, and has had the most success with so far, has been the stem cell transplant. They take and collect the stem cells of the patient, if they can. If they can't do that, then they try to find a donor who matches the patient. That's the most serious one because of the rejection aspect. As long as they can collect stem cells from the patient, there is an excellent chance of being successful.

In my case, they were able to collect 70 million stem cells the first time they made the collection. Now, that's an awful lot of cells. The procedure requires that you have high dosage chemotherapy four times, and then they make the stem cell transplant. The transplant is not surgery; it's simply a killing of the blood cells in the bone marrow and then giving you back the stem cells they collected in the blood through intravenous injections.

It's rare, it's tough, and a lot of people have problems with it. Fortunately for me, I did not have any kind of problem with the collection, with the chemotherapy, with anything that I've taken. I have been in remission since January of 2001. And everything is just going super good as far as I'm concerned.

At some point in time, my myeloma will come back. It may come back in five years, ten years, or two months from now. There's really no way to know when it will come back, but it will.

The other thing I got lucky with (and, when I say luck, I really believe it is) is Thalidomide, which is that high-powered drug that was developed in England for morning sickness about thirty or forty years ago. As you may remember, Thalidomide was a disaster. It was the cause of many birth defects and was outlawed for pregnant women because it cuts off the blood supply to developing cells. The developing cells in the body are basically creating new babies or cancer.

Cancer research centers all over the country said, "Well, if it cuts off the blood supply for developing cells, why would it not cut off the blood supply for cancer?" Dr. Barlogie started using it in Little Rock in 1998, and it's been very, very successful at putting patients in remission. It's high-dosage; it's heavy. Thalidomide is very, very expensive at ten to twelve dollars a tablet. Initially, I was put on eight tablets per day. Physically, I couldn't handle that much. It made me feel like I had palsy. I was shaky and my legs burned. They reduced it to four, which I could handle. Right now I'm on one per day and don't have any side effects.

My three keys to cancer survival are: One, have a strong faith in God; Two, have a positive attitude; And three, stay busy. There's not an hour that goes by in my life that I don't realize that I have cancer. And as quickly as I realize that, I think about something else. That's been my game plan. Fortunately, my work allows me to do that. But you can't get away from realizing that you have the disease. You just can't get away from it. It's going to be there. While all of the three survival keys are important, the first, having a strong faith in God, is the one you must have to really make it work.

"Beating cancer has a lot to do with your mental state."

> — *Eddie Van Halen—cancer*
> *of the tongue, rock star*

"The attitude of the cancer patient is vitally important. A patient who is ready to help fight and work with his or her physician has a better chance of recovery than one who is very passive."

> — *Peter K. Vogt, Ph.D.,*
> *Head, Division of Oncovirology,*
> *The Scripps Research Institute*

"I have a positive attitude, which I think plays a great part in anyone's recovery. And I urge anyone over fifty to get a colonoscopy to detect colon cancer. It's a very simple test— and it can save your life."

> — *Rod Roddy—colon cancer,*
> The Price is Right *announcer*

Bob Williams—metastasized squamous
Sixty-two years old—Anderson, South Carolina
Retired, volunteers for Habitat For Humanity

Metastasized squamous can affect any moist area of your body. It can go to your kidneys, your bladder, your lungs, your throat. Mine was, they thought, somewhere in my sinuses. Somewhere just below my eyes, but above my collarbone. They had to do a radical neck dissection where they removed the mastoid muscle on the left side, cut all the nerves, and took out everything they could find. I had a lymph node that swelled. That's how they knew what it was. Then I had thirty-seven radiation treatments and four months of chemotherapy.

I did the radiation and the chemo at the same time, and was I ever a sick puppy. I lost forty-four pounds. I was gray, and I couldn't eat because my throat was so blistered. I was in the hospital for seven days; and they pumped chemo through me for seven days solid, night and day, twenty-four hours a day. Then I'd go down to radiation, where they fastened my face down to the table, under the machine, so I wouldn't move.

They had this mask I had to put on. It was very claustrophobic and, of course, my chemo machine was over to my right pumping away. I was afraid I was going to start throwing up and choke on it. But they were always listening. It was very quiet.

The radiation's just warm, but I got blistered, my face burned purple. Chemo just makes you really, really nauseated; it doesn't hurt you. It's refrigerated until it's cold, so your body temperature is very cold all the time.

One time I got to the point where I wanted to stop the chemo. I just couldn't take it any longer. But it wasn't because I wanted to die; that was never an option. I needed to live. I had to be there to take care of my mother during her health crisis. Of course, whatever the Lord had in mind for me was what was going to happen.

Every time I was in the hospital, somebody died on the oncology floor. I would hear on the loud speaker, "Code blue." That was the call for the crash cart. The nurses were so nice, they would come in and sit on my bed and say, "Don't worry, it's not the same as yours."

I was really close with a man across the hall. His wife and daughter would come and visit me in my room. He had lung cancer, but he didn't make it. That really hurt, but like I said, dying was never an option for me.

One of my side effects, beside the fact that I have no saliva, is that the chemo caused the uric acid in my kidneys to crystallize and I have a lot of kidney stones now.

I look in the mirror and say, "What happened to you, you old fart?" But I'm still here. I don't look like it, but I'm still here. But either way, I have to attribute whatever success I've had with cancer to faith and to prayer, and dealing with it in that way.

"The Lord gave me the strength to do it, and I think that's the answer for anyone. I wanted to quit the chemo after the second session, but my oncologist said, 'No, you're not going to do that.' He has a really deep voice. I understand the Lord does, also."

— *Bob Williams*

Derek Werner—melanoma
Forty-four years of age—Beijing, China
U.S. diplomat

Everyone deals with cancer and life-threatening diseases so differently. My sister's husband got melanoma the year before I did (1998) and died three months later, so it really hit home when I was diagnosed with it, too. My brother-in-law was very private and didn't let my sister tell anyone about it. My parents found out the day he died, as did I. He finally told his own mother the night before he died. It was really tough on my sister. It was not the way I dealt with it.

I am very much a realist in all things in life. When I found out I had melanoma, I told my oncology surgeon that I wanted to know exactly what was going on and did not want anything sugar-coated. That was in July of 1999, and he told me it was possible that I might not make the millennium. My response was half in jest and half masking my fear: "I have to make the millennium, we already have an invitation to a great party!" He countered that was exactly the kind of attitude to have. He said some patients just roll over and basically die when they find out they have cancer.

For me, it was therapeutic to learn as much as I could about melanoma through the Internet, and through my doctor, who is now a good friend. I let friends know I would not seek sympathy, but I wanted to learn from others who had had it. I was going to Bethesda Medical Center (where the President goes) and after gaining considerable knowledge, I felt like I was getting the best treatment possible. My surgeon tells me he wishes his residents knew as much about melanoma as I do. I always have ten or fifteen new questions with every follow-up.

It was very comforting to feel like I was doing everything I could. I realize I could die in the next year, but at least I'm doing everything I can to stay alive because I love life! Another friend from college, a neurological surgeon, told me that he wasn't a cancer specialist but thought my positive attitude toward life could be very beneficial. He said he has known people with cancer who had a great prognosis but died because they just gave up, while others, with not so hot a prognosis, lived forever. That helped make me even more positive on life.

My wife Jennie and I learned I had cancer while in Washington, D.C., two days before we were moving to Bogota, Colombia. It turns out the surgery I needed couldn't be done by the surgeon I wanted for a month. We could have moped around Washington waiting but instead, we decided to move to Bogota as planned and then come back for my surgery.

We had a blast going to welcome parties. We went on a neat trip to a colonial Colombian village, and we were so busy that month that we didn't have time to worry too much about my upcoming surgery. I had what is called a wide margin excision. They took out about an inch deep and then stretched my skin and sewed me back up. I was lucky I didn't have to have a skin graft.

I also had a sentinel lymph node biopsy. They removed a couple of lymph nodes under my left arm to see if the cancer had spread there. Based on the biopsy (95 percent accuracy), it had not spread, thank God! I was and am in pretty decent shape and was told that helped a lot in my quick recovery from having a big chunk taken out of my back. The only exercise I held off on for a long time was push-ups. The doctors said to wait a month. It took about three weeks after that to get back to the normal 200 push-ups that I do every other day.

I didn't have any more treatments. With melanoma there really aren't any effective treatments at this point—radiation and chemo don't seem to do much for it. There are clinical trials going on with different drugs, but nothing works well thus far. I went in for check-ups every three months, now every six months, to look for new melanomas.

We won't ever really know that everything is 100 percent perfect but if I get through five years, I have an 80 percent chance of living to my normal life expectancy. The dermatologist in Beijing, China, where we now live, thought I had another melanoma this past May and took five biopsies (she didn't think the other four were melanoma but she wanted to be sure) and, fortunately, they all came up benign. I don't think about my melanoma a lot, but I'm very open to talking about it with others who have cancer. For me, staying positive and, even more than ever, living life to the fullest, is paramount.

My advice (at least to realists) is to learn as much as you can about your disease and get second opinions so you really know what your options are. Manage your own medical care as much as possible. I would also say that it is good to go on living as you have been as much as possible (that is, if you are happy with your life!), stay positive, and savor every day. This probably sounds like a bunch of clichés, but I truly believe what I'm saying.

"The cancer made me realize I had to be a great deal more appreciative, to tell people that I love them. To be quick to say to someone, 'That's a good job, wonderful.' Life is too short to waste it on nastiness."

— *Archbishop Desmond Tutu—prostate cancer*

"We are closer to curing cancer than President Kennedy was to success when he pledged to put a man on the moon. I feel affiliated with that frontier of hope."

> — *Rob Lowe,*
> *television and movie actor, whose grand-*
> *mother and great-grandmother died of*
> *breast cancer. His father is in remission*
> *from non-Hodgkin's lymphoma.*

"On a good day, I went to a wedding brunch and was relaxing on a sofa chatting with old friends when a woman I had not seen since my disease was diagnosed as peritoneal cancer spied me from across the room. She rushed over, kissed me on the cheek, and standing erect with her finger pointing to the ceiling pronounced, 'Harry is waiting for you up there!' The entire room immediately retreated into shocked silence. Her husband, Harry, had died the year before. All I could manage was a flippant, 'I hope Harry has a long wait.' "

> — *Barbara Gamarekian—peritoneal*
> *cancer (cancer of the membrane*
> *lining the walls of the abdominal cavity*
> *and enclosing the viscera), former*
> *reporter for* The New York Times

The Last Word

The thing about getting cancer is that, perhaps for the first time, you start thinking about your own life span. When you do that, cancer forces you to change—for good or for bad—depending upon how you handle it. You suddenly realize there is no guarantee of time.

Cancer survivors are well aware that life is just today. It is now. Go live it.

" I firmly believe life is not how you start, it's how you finish.

I want to be a good finisher."

— *Brian Doyle—late-stage leukemia
(in full remission), second baseman,
hit .438 in 1978 World Series
for winning New York Yankees*

Cancer Camp Directory

Hole In The Wall Gang Camp
555 Long Wharf Drive
New Haven, Connecticut, 06511
Executive director: Jim Canton
(203) 772-0522

The Imus Ranch
P.O. Box 250
Ribera, New mexico, 87560
Ranch coordinator: Samantha Imus
(505) 421-IMUS

Camp Oochigeas
66 Sinclair Avenue, East
Suite 201
Toronto, Ontario M4T1N5
Director: Maija Bradshaw
(416) 961-6624

Silver Lining Ranch
1490 Ute Avenue
Aspen, Colorado, 81611
Cofounder: Andrea Jaeger
(970) 925-9540

Index

Abraham, Robert, 16–19, *137*
Allan, Mary, 123–124
Armstrong, Lance, *31*, *168*

Baker, Dusty, *167*
Baylor, Don, *178*
Benz, Jr., Dr. Edward J., *12*
Bernstein, Dr. Joel, 30
Bickers, Bennie, 155–156, *165*
Bradshaw, Maija, 95–96
Burroughs, Gene, 157–158
Bush, President George W., *114*

Camp Oochigeas, 95–96, 191
Canton, Jim, 83–86
Carter, Betsy, *130*
Channing, Carol, *171*
Condren, Tom, 181–182
Connally, Nellie B., 109–112
Connolly, Denise, 121–122
Cooper, David, *154*
Cox, Dave, *163*, *169*
Crawford, Dr. David, 8–9, 134
Cunningham, Randall "Duke", *20*

Davidson, Elizabeth, 44–45
Davidson, Dr. Nancy, *102*
Dawson, Len and Linda, 149–151
Dick, Anne, 129
Doren, Kim, *117*
Douglas, Briten, 67–69
Douglas, Corinna, 63
Doyle, Brian, *190*

Eck, Keith, 175–177
Ellsworth, Doris, *25*, *50*
Espy, Bill, 159–160
Eszterhas, Joe, *82*

Floyd, Raymond, *166*
Foster, Dr. Chris, *164*
Friend, Dr. Stephen, 11–12, 65, 102

Gamarekian, Barbara, 189
Geppi-Aikens, Diane, *180*
Giuliani, Rudy, *145*, *154*, *178*
Glaser, Ellie, *23*, 49–50
Goodman, Dr. Cole, 57–58
Goodman, Dorothy, 56
Goodman, Dr. R.C., 55–56
Goodman, Wyndal, 58–61

Hall, Dr. Richard, ix, *36*, *169*
Hamilton, Scott, *3*
Hodgens, Dr. David, 15, 100–101, *160*
Hole In The Wall Gang Camp, 83–88, 191

Imus Ranch, The, 93–94, 191
Imus, Samantha, 93–94

Jaeger, Andrea, 89–92
Jenkins, Adriana, *124*
Johnson, Arte, 53
Jones, Ann Williams, *126*
Jones, Charlie, *19*, *54*, *141*

Krant, Dr. Stephen, 170–171
Kunsel, Minerva, 125–126

Leverant, "Izzy", 127
Lowe, Rob, *189*
Lythgoe, Wendy, 32–33

Marks, Dr. Paul, 5, 173
Marshall, Jr., Vern, 42–43
Marshall, Sr.,Vern, 42–43
McGraw, Tug, *61*
McTierman, Dr. Anne, *130*
Mendelsohn, Dr. John, 2–3, 21–22, 64, 133, 169
Merkins, Linda, 40–41, 128
Miller, Guy, 70–71
Morariu, Corina, *33*
Murchison III, Clint, 161

Newman, Paul, 87–88

Osbourne, Sharon, 62

Palmer, Arnold, 166
Potts, Bill, 146–148
Press, Ben, *164*

Reina, Ron, 179–180
Ritt, Dr. Don, 26–27
Roddy, Rod, *183*
Rosenthal, Maryann, 24–25, 51–52, 66, 174

Schilling, Shonda, *48*
Schimmer, Ernie and Maria, 79–81
Schmidt, Vicki, *27*
Seabolt, Alden, 74
Seabolt, Steve, 75
Shea, Dr. Peder, *10*
Shephard, Joy, 99, 103–108
Sherrill, Dr. Jim, 34–35
Shively, Dr. Harold, 46–47
Silver Lining Ranch, 89–92, 191

Simpson, Kurt, 37–39
Smith, Steve, 142–144
Speer, Carol, 76
Speer, Kyle, 76

Thorton, Jennifer, 77–78
Torre, Joe, *167*
Trombold, Dr. John, 28, *29*
Tutu, Archbishop Desmond, *188*

Van Halen, Eddie, *183*
Veneman, Ann, 113–114
Vogt, Peter, 6, *14*, *183*
von Eschenbach, Dr. Andrew, 13, *14*, *101*

Waitley, Denis, 138–141
Wahman, Dr. Gerald, *36*, 135–137, *173*
Waldman, Suzyn, 115–117
Wallace, Dr. Anne, 7, 98–99, 172
Walsh, Dr. Patrick, 4, *36*, 132, *165*
Werner, Derek, 186–188
Williams, Bob, 184–185
Wolford, Ballard, 72–73
Wolford, "C.B.", 72
Wolford, Eddie Dean, 73
Wolford, Faye, 72

York, Herbert, 162

About the Authors

Charlie Jones is the *New York Times* best-selling author of *What Makes Winners Win*. He is a graduate of the University of Arkansas School of Law with a juris doctor degree. He recently received the Arkansas Distinguished Alumnus Award, and presented the commencement speech. Charlie is also one of the most versatile sportscasters in history. He has broadcast twenty-seven different sports around the world, including three Summer Olympic Games. For four decades he broadcast the NFL on network television. Charlie is a Pro Football Hall of Fame inductee, a member of the Arkansas Sports Hall of Fame, and the winner of an Emmy and a Cine Golden Eagle. His PSA is now 0.1.

Kim Doren is an avid world traveler whose diverse experiences have included working as a jillaroo in Outback Australia, teaching English in inner city Washington, D.C. and directing advertising and marketing for Cobra Golf. A graduate of Stanford University, Kim is an accomplished athlete and photographer. She is active in several non-profit organizations, enjoys giving motivational speeches, and loves sharing time with her five nieces. Kim lives in La Jolla, California.

Charlie Jones and Kim Doren are co-authors of *You Go Girl!: The Winning Way*; *Be the Ball: A Golf Book for the Mind*; *Game, Set, Match: A Tennis Book for the Mind*; *That's Outside My Boat: Letting Go of What You Can't Control*; and *If Winning Were Easy, Everyone Would Do It*.